Insights on Antimicrobial Peptides

Edited by Shymaa Enany, Jorge Masso-Silva and Anna Savitskaya

Published in London, United Kingdom

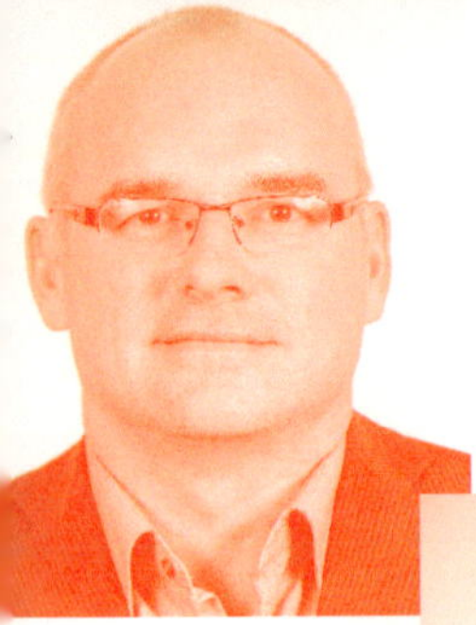

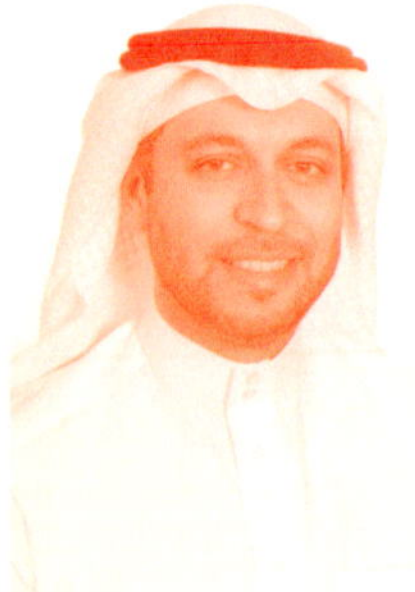

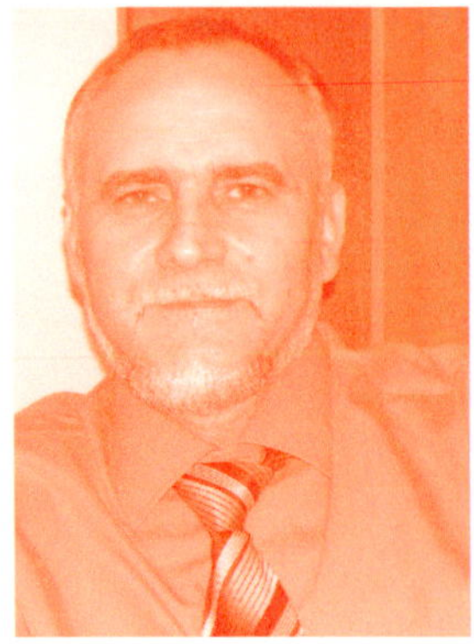

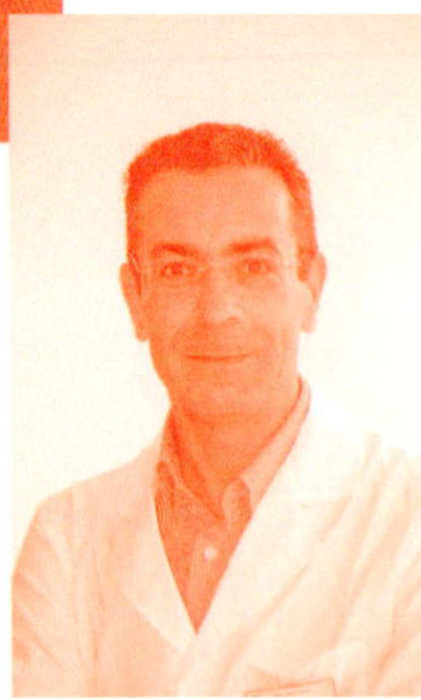

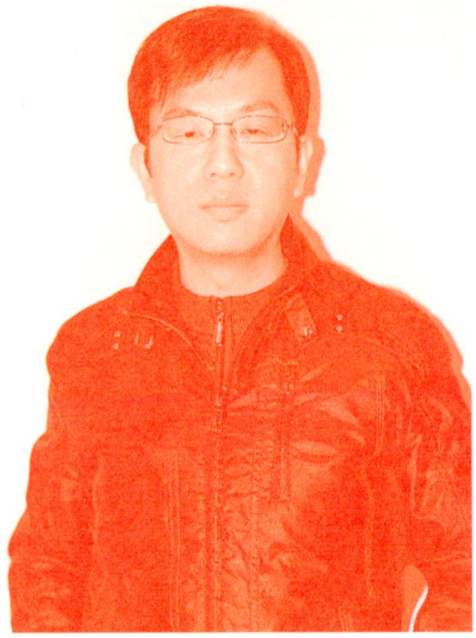

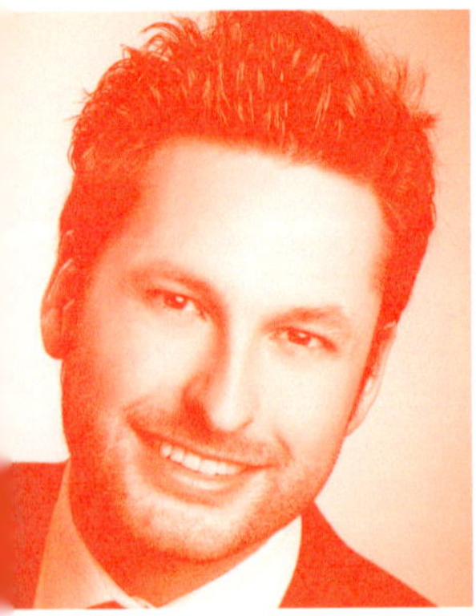

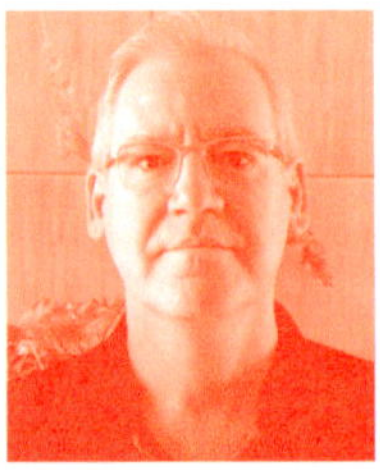

IntechOpen

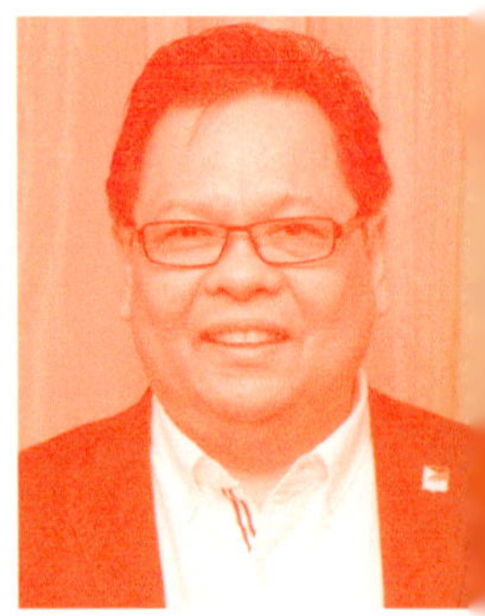

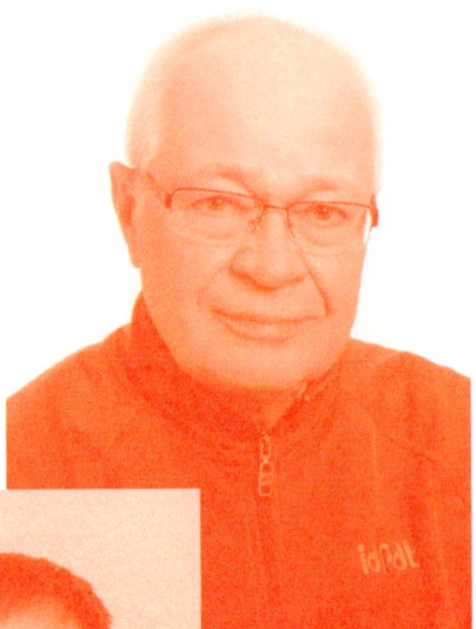

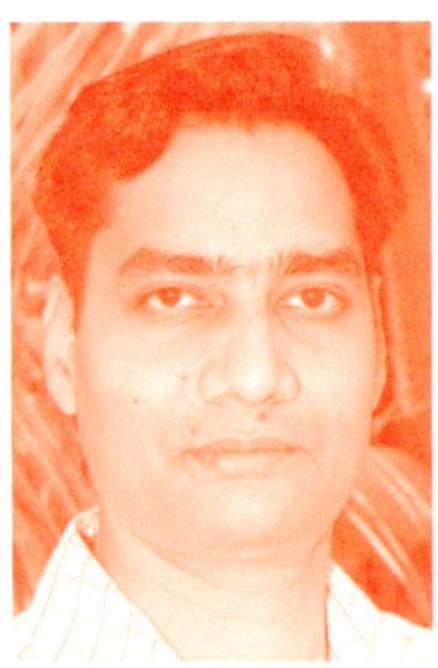

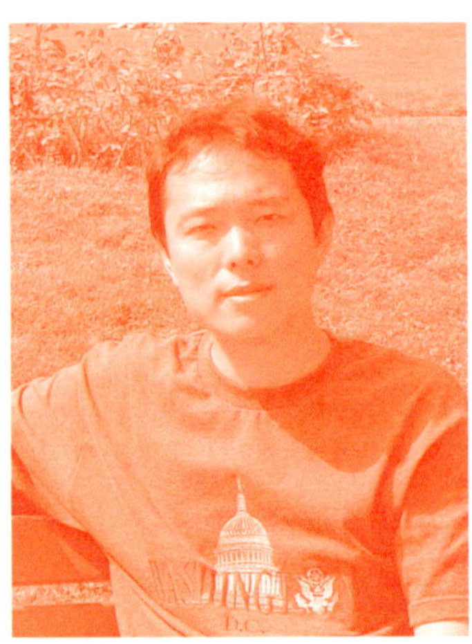

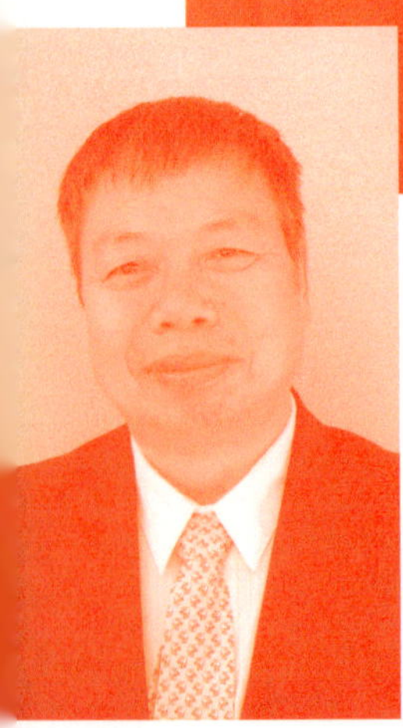

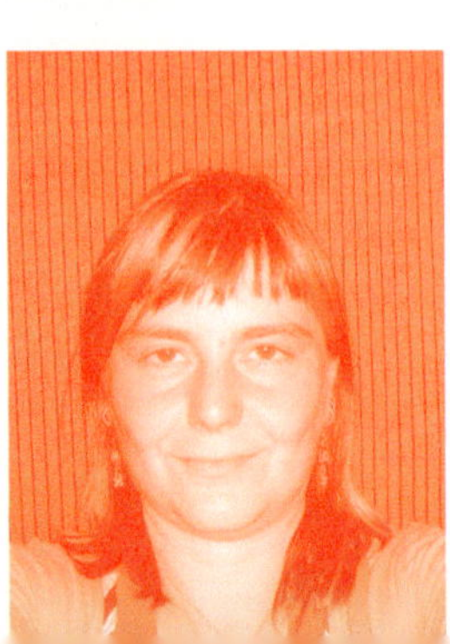

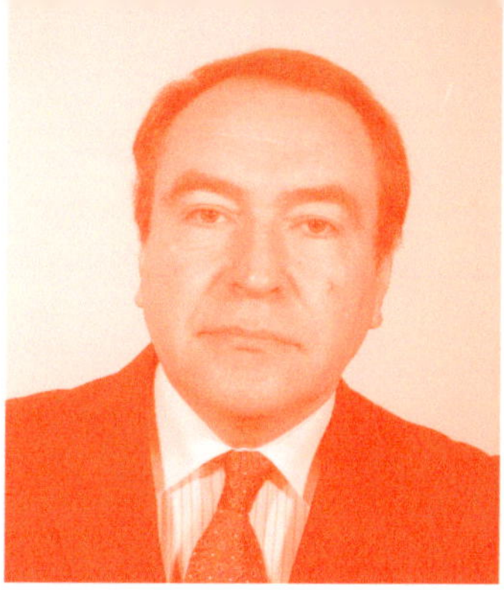
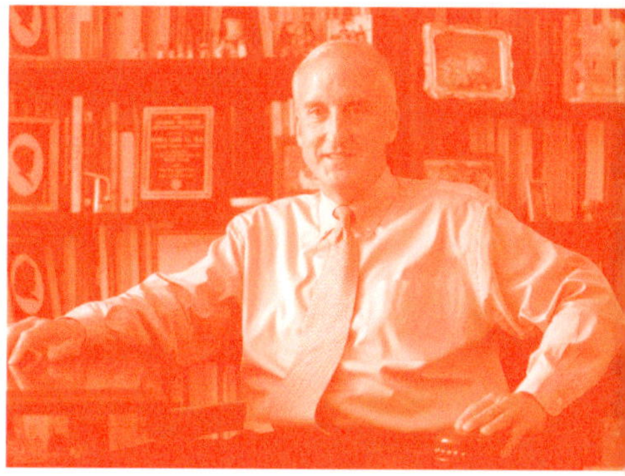
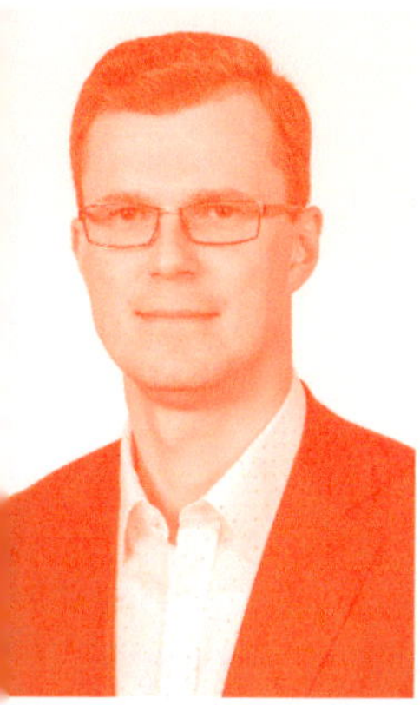
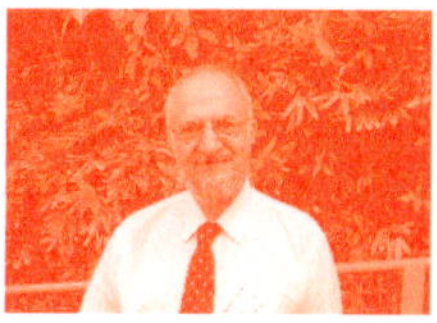
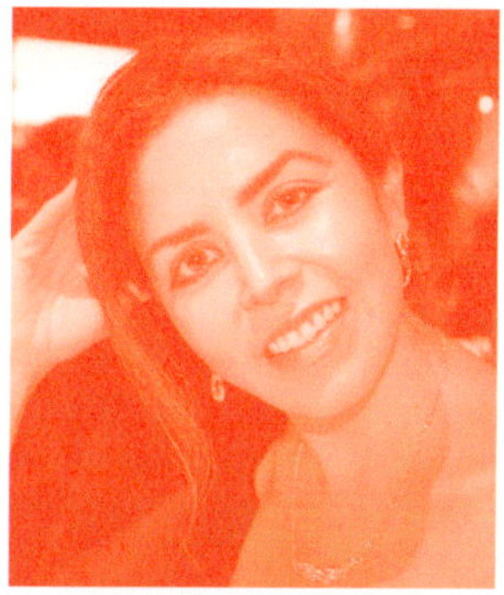

Supporting open minds since 2005

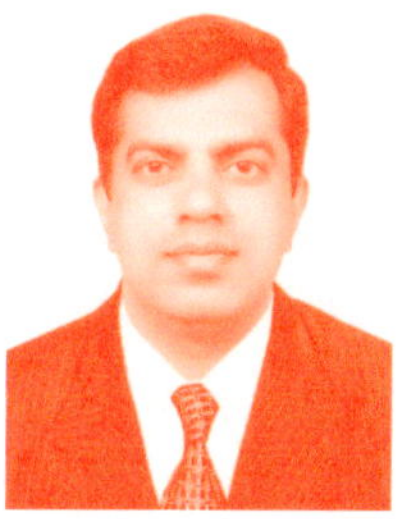
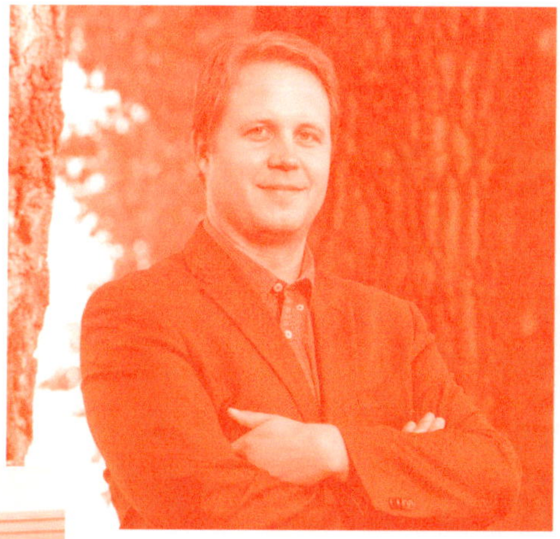
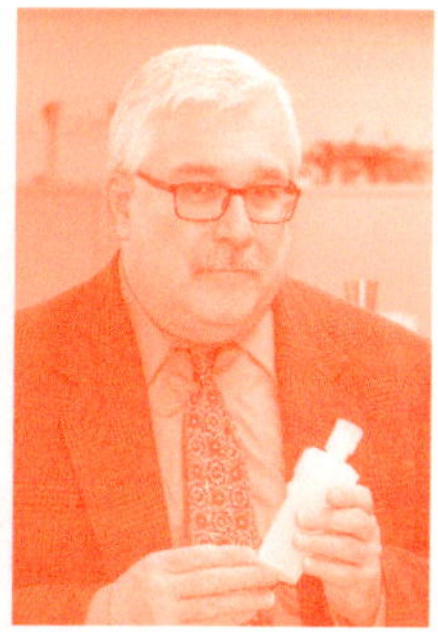
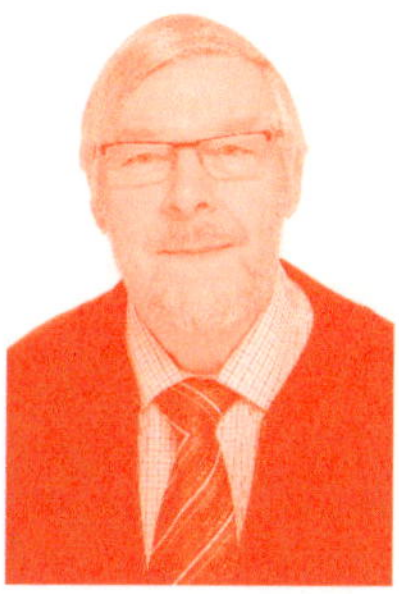
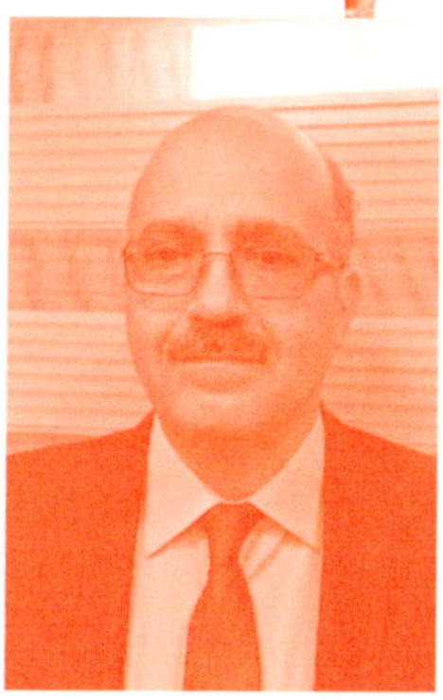
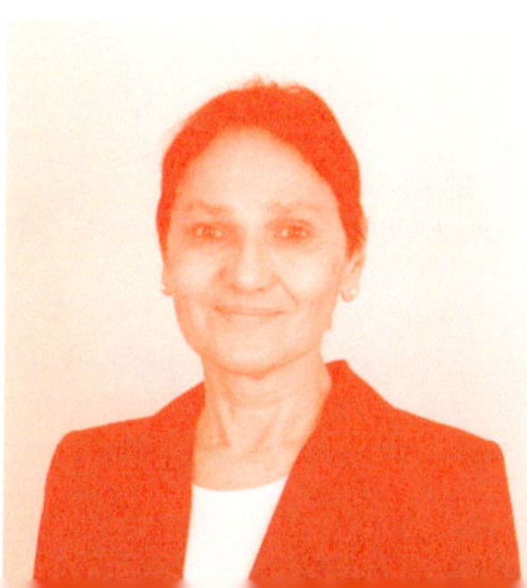
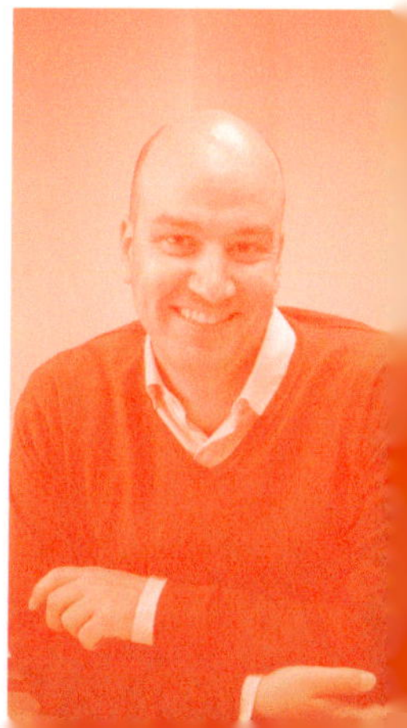

Insights on Antimicrobial Peptides
http://dx.doi.org/10.5772/intechopen.95183
Edited by Shymaa Enany, Jorge Masso-Silva and Anna Savitskaya

Contributors
Miquel Blasco, Diego Jáuregui, Santiago Mafla, Haamid Bashir, Sabhiya Majid Majid, Mohammad Hayat Bhat, Rajaian Pushpabai Rajesh, Grace Vanathi M, Geert Baggerman, Eline Berghmans, Sangeeta Singh, Tanu Singh, Princy Choudhary, Awatef Ouertani, Amor Mosbah, Ameur Cherif, Salvatore De-Simone, Karyne Rangel, Shymaa Enany, Jorge Adrian Masso-Silva, Anna Savitskaya

First published in London, United Kingdom, 2022 by IntechOpen
IntechOpen is the global imprint of INTECHOPEN LIMITED, registered in England and Wales, registration number: 11086078, 5 Princes Gate Court, London, SW7 2QJ, United Kingdom
Printed in Croatia

British Library Cataloguing-in-Publication Data
A catalogue record for this book is available from the British Library

Additional hard and PDF copies can be obtained from orders@intechopen.com

Insights on Antimicrobial Peptides
Edited by Shymaa Enany, Jorge Masso-Silva and Anna Savitskaya
p. cm.
Print ISBN 978-1-83969-713-5
Online ISBN 978-1-83969-714-2
eBook (PDF) ISBN 978-1-83969-715-9

For EU product safety concerns:
IN TECH d.o.o., Prolaz Marije Krucifikse Kozulić 3, 51000 Rijeka, Croatia, info@intechopen.com or visit our website at intechopen.com.

Meet the editors

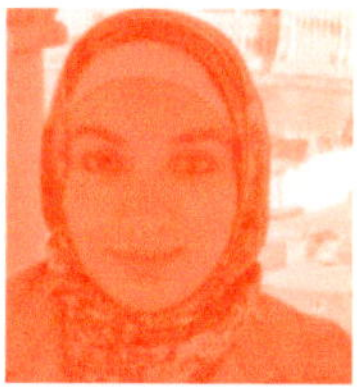

Dr. Shymaa Enany is an Associate Professor of Microbiology, at Suez Canal University, Egypt, and is currently working at Armed Forces College of Medicine, Egypt. She received her Ph.D. from the School of Medical Sciences, Niigata University, Japan. She completed her post-doctoral studies in the United States and Japan. Dr. Enany was one of the first Arab scientists to apply bacterial proteomic techniques to reveal good markers for microbes spreading in the community. She has received many awards for her scientific contributions, including the 2021 International Science Council Award for Early Career Scientist in Africa, the 2019 Egyptian state encouragement prize for women in the field of health and pharmaceutical sciences, and the 2018 World Academy of Sciences Young Arab Scientist Prize in Medical Sciences.

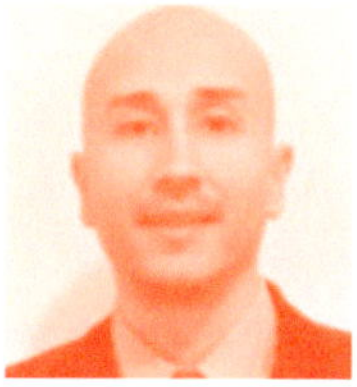

Dr. Jorge A. Masso-Silva is interested in immunology and how our immune system protects us from pathogens. He obtained his master's degree in Biotechnology from Centro de Investigaciones Biologicas del Noroeste, Mexico in 2007. He obtained his Ph.D. in Biomedical Science from Rutgers University, USA, in 2012 with research on innate and adaptive immune responses. Dr. Masso-Silva worked for the Federal Government in Mexico and is a member of the National System of Investigators in Mexico. Currently, he is a postdoc in the Division of Pulmonary Critical Care and Sleep, Section Chief of Pulmonary Critical Care Medicine, University of California at San Diego, USA.

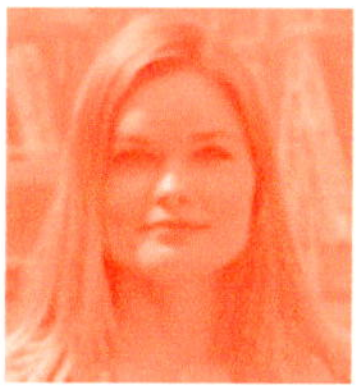

Dr. Anna Savitskaya, Ph.D., is a senior researcher at the Institute of Bioorganic Chemistry, Russian Academy of Science, Moscow. Her research interests include microbiology, molecular genetics, the use of microorganisms as producers of target proteins, and analysis of intracellular protein interaction. She obtained a Ph.D. from Niigata University in 2012. Since 2008, she has been enrolled in a Ph.D. course at the Department of Chemical Technologies of Wood and Biotechnology, Siberian State University of Science and Technology. In the same year, she began working as a junior researcher at the biotechnology laboratory of the Krasnoyarsk Agriculture Research Institute. In 2011, Dr. Savitskaya completed an internship at the University of Ottawa, Canada.

Contents

Preface XI

Chapter 1 1
Introductory Chapter: Antimicrobial Peptides – Prodigious Therapeutic Strategies
by Jorge Masso-Silva, Anna Savitskaya and Shymaa Enany

Chapter 2 7
Anti-Microbial Peptides: The Importance of Structure-Function Analysis in the Design of New AMPs
by Awatef Ouertani, Amor Mosbah and Ameur Cherif

Chapter 3 23
Antimicrobial Peptides: Mechanism of Action
by Tanu Singh, Princy Choudhary and Sangeeta Singh

Chapter 4 43
Antimicrobial Peptides Derived from Ascidians and Associated Cyanobacteria
by Rajaian Pushpabai Rajesh and Grace Vanathi M

Chapter 5 69
Molecular Pathogenesis of Inflammatory Cytokines in Insulin Resistance Diabetes Mellitus
by Haamid Bashir, Mohammad Hayat Bhat and Sabhiya Majid

Chapter 6 87
Mass Spectrometry (Imaging) for Detection and Identification of Cyclic AMPs: Focus on Human Neutrophil Peptides (HNPs)
by Eline Berghmans and Geert Baggerman

Chapter 7 105
Cloning and Identification System of *Apis mellifera* Melittin cDNA in *Escherichia coli*
by Diego Jáuregui, Miquel Blasco and Santiago Mafla

Chapter 8 113
Peptides with Therapeutic Potential against *Acinetobacter baumanii* Infections
by Karyne Rangel and Salvatore Giovanni De-Simone

Preface

Microorganisms are ubiquitous and play an important but "bifacial" role in the existence of plants, animals, and humans. Some microorganisms are necessary for maintaining vital functions but may play a negative role and lead to infectious diseases and even death. Thus, all existing species must protect themselves from excess colonization of microorganisms that can cause infection and death. The immune system defends the organism against different types of infections. Antimicrobial peptides (AMPs) are an important part of the innate immune system of different organisms living in nature. Unfortunately, the immune system cannot always defeat the infection. Infectious diseases were an enormous problem in the past. Before the discovery of antibiotics, extracts of herbs and plants and chemical compounds were used as therapies for infectious diseases. Everything changed with the discovery of penicillin, which marked the start of the "antibiotic era." Antibiotics were determined to be "miracle drugs" and intensively used in medicine for the successful treatment of bacterial infection. However, this intensive usage in human and veterinary medicine, sometimes as a preventive step, has led to drug resistance.

Microorganisms are good at adapting to different stress conditions and have different mechanisms of antibiotic resistance such as alteration of membrane permeability, enzymatic degradation of antibiotics, modification of bacterial proteins that are antimicrobial targets, and active efflux. Modern medicine is impossible without antibiotics, but conclusions of the "antibiotic era" aren't optimistic. Global antibiotic usage led to the development of superbugs, and the number of resistant bacteria and multidrug-resistant (MDR) bacteria is rapidly increasing. As such, we still have problems with infectious disease treatment despite an arsenal of antibiotics, many of which have become ineffective against modern (resistant) microorganisms.

Another problem with modern antibacterial treatment is that we currently use antibiotics discovered more than three decades ago. A new antibiotic is necessary, but unfortunately, the development of new antibiotics is costly, takes years, and is an unprofitable process for pharmaceutical companies.

This book presents a comprehensive overview of AMPs with potential for medical use. The AMPs described are isolated from different sources, such as ascidians, cyanobacteria, frogs, and more.

Chapter by Rajesh and Vanathi describes the structure and mechanism of action of bioactive peptides derived from ascidians and associated cyanobacteria that are structurally unique and have antibacterial, antifungal, and anticancer activity. Chapter by Rangel and De Simone discusses peptides from different sources that are active against the ESKAPE group of antibiotic-resistant bacteria, especially anti-Acinetobacter peptides, as *A. baumannii* has emerged as a highly troublesome nosocomial pathogen revealing drug-resistant (DR), MDR, extensively drug-resistant (XDR), and pan-drug-resistant (PDR) phenotypes. Chapter by Ouertani et al. discusses bacteriocins, which are bacterial AMPs. The chapter focuses on the structure-function relationship and mechanism of action of AMPs.

This timely book presents the current situation of AMPs as an emerging group of therapeutic agents. It is a useful resource for clinicians, researchers, technicians, scientists, and students. Finally, we would like to thank all the contributing authors for their time and original research.

Shymaa Enany
Faculty of Pharmacy,
Department of Microbiology and Immunology,
Suez Canal University,
Ismailia, Egypt

Jorge Masso-Silva
Division of Pulmonary Critical Care and Sleep,
Section Chief of Pulmonary Critical Care Medicine,
University of California at San Diego,
San Diego, USA

Anna Savitskaya
Institute of Bioorganic Chemistry of Russian Academy of Science,
Moscow, Russian Federation

Chapter 1

Introductory Chapter: Antimicrobial Peptides – Prodigious Therapeutic Strategies

Jorge Masso-Silva, Anna Savitskaya and Shymaa Enany

1. Introduction

Antimicrobial peptides (AMPs) exist in all living things, from unicellular to more complex multicellular organisms [1]. They are at the frontline of defense against microbial pathogens [1, 2]. In less complex organisms, AMPs represent a major part of their arsenal against detrimental organisms, and on the other hand, more evolved organisms have a wider repertoire of biological weapons against these detrimental organisms [3, 4]. AMPs are typically amphipatic small peptides usually under 50 amino acids with a net positive charge at physiological pH [5].

Although AMP_S were described for the first time in the 1960s, it was until 1980s were the AMP called cecropin was identified and characterized from a moth [6]. Since then, many AMPs have been identified in all different taxa from microorganisms, plants, invertebrates, and vertebrates [3]. In vertebrates, AMPs have been widely characterized in all different phylogenetic classes, from fish to mammals [3, 7]. Currently, over 2600 AMPs have been identified, and most of them in eukaryotes [8].

In vertebrates, AMPs can be expressed in different compartments, from the skin to specific cells within internal organs and blood. Thus, their action can be found throughout the whole body, and this is where the relevance of AMPs relies on for the protection of the host.

In addition, in other taxa, gene duplication has been an important factor for the evolution of AMPs. In plants, for example, gene duplication has led to the creation of large families of AMPs. For example, in plants such as *Arabidopsis* and *Medicago* up to 300 different sequences of defensin and defensin-like have been found [4, 9].

Although for many years it was thought that the main role of AMPs was the killing of pathogens to resolve infections, now it is known that the variety of functions of AMPs ranges from direct antimicrobial activity to a wide range of immunomodulatory mechanisms, hence their importance in host defenses. In infections, depending on the phase of infection, their immunomodulatory activity can be either pro- or anti-inflammatory [5]. Initially, the scientific community focused their research on the potential of AMPs as therapeutics due to their antibiotic properties, although now it is well established that AMPs have more roles beyond that and are playing a key role in immunity [5].

2. Classes of antimicrobial peptides

Despite that most AMPs are amphipathic, they can differ significantly in sequence and structure. To simplify their classification due to their wide diversity, AMPs have been classified based on (1) source, (2) activity, (3) structural characteristics, and

 IntechOpen

(4) amino acid-rich species [10]. Based on source, they can be divided into mammals, amphibians, microorganisms, and insects. In mammals and vertebrates in general, the two main classes of AMPs are defensins and cathelicidins, which are produced as prepropepides that required site-specific cleavage to reach their mature and active form [1, 11]. Based on their activity, they can be divided into 18 categories according to the ADP3 database, which can be summarized as antibacterial, antiviral, antifungal, antiparasitic, antihuman immunodeficiency virus (HIV), and antitumor peptides [10]. Based on structure, they are divided into four structures due to their tridimensional conformation: α-helical linear peptides, peptides with β-sheet forming disulfide bridges, with both α-helix and β-sheet peptides, and peptides with extended flexible loop structures [3, 4, 10]. In addition, cyclic AMPs with more complex topologies are also reported [10]. Finally, based on amino acid rich context, they are divided into proline-rich, tryptophan- and arginine-rich, histidine-rich, and glycine-rich antimicrobial peptides [10].

3. Mechanism of action

In terms of their mechanism of action, bacteria membranes have been a key model to assess direct antimicrobial activity, which are initiated through electrostatic interaction from the cationic nature of AMPs and the negative charge of bacterial membranes due to the anionic lipids (lipopolysaccharides in Gram-negative batceria and teichoic acid in Gram-positive bacteria) [5]. This results in poor interaction with membranes of cells from plants, invertebrates, and vertebrates. There are four different models in which AMPs can interact with bacterial cells, leading to leakage of the cell content and further cell death. These models are 1) aggregate, 2) toroidal pore, 3) barrel stave, and 4) carpet [3]. Amphipatic AMPs possess amino acids with hydrophilic and hydrophobic side chains at opposite sides, which allow them to interact with membranes of bacteria that are negatively charged [5].

In the case of viruses, several mechanisms of action have been identified, such as the destabilization of viral envelope on contact (damaging virions and thus diminishing their infectivity), decreasing viral replication and/or binding of viral capsid (preventing entry of the viral genome), aggregation of viral particles, and immunomodulation [3, 5]. For antifungal purposes, it has been reported that AMPs effects range from the membrane effects to impairment in mitochondrial function [5, 12, 13]. It is important to consider that fungi can form biofilms, which are highly resistant to antifungals, which challenge even more the identification and development of biofilm-forming fungi [14].

Besides the direct microbicidal activity, immunomodulatory function of AMPs has been of a key focus from more recent years. The studies have define a diverse range of immunomodulatory function that is highly complex and seems to be dependent on the environmental stimuli, cell and tissue type, interaction with different cellular receptors, and the concentration of the peptides [3, 5, 15]. AMPs can interact with both membrane-associated and intracellular receptors, and they can cause alterations of several signaling pathways and engagement with different transcription factors [2, 15].

3.1 Therapeutic use

Since the discovery of AMPs, a significant part of their research has been focused on their potential therapeutic use. Currently, with the raise of antibiotic resistance, there is an increasing challenge for human health. The development of more efficient antibiotics has decreased as compared with previous years, and along with the abuse of the use of these antibiotics, we have created the conditions to originate bacteria super resistant of widely used antibiotics, which has generated incredible economical and health burden [5, 16, 17]. This phenomenon has also occurred with fungi, whose incidence still affects millions of individuals every year [18]. Thus, there has been an urgent need for the generation of new antibiotics with low potential for the generation of resistance.

As mentioned before, due to the mechanism of action of AMPs that rely mostly in electrostatic interactions and not in specific targets, it was thought that it is unlikely that microbes can become resistant to AMPs. Thus, this feature of AMPs have attracted investigators and industry to study them with the goal to be use as therapeutics against pathogenic bacteria mostly, although some studies have address this approach against fungi [19], viruses [20], and parasites [21]. However, there is evidence of resistance to direct killing by AMP and related synthetic analogs by multiple mechanisms from bacteria [22–24]. Although in consequence of the generation of resistance to AMPs, there is a cost in fitness for infectivity leading to impaired survival and pathogencity *in vivo* [25]. Thus, there is a current area of research in AMPs focusing more in harnessing the immunomodulatory actions of AMPs in order to enhance host immune responses rather that direct killing of the pathogen [5]. Moreover, their synergistic potential as adjuvants with other antimicrobial compounds is another area of interest [26].

The use of natural AMPs has shown poor viability due to the relatively high concentrations necessary at which these AMPs have to be affective, which often leads to cytotoxicity [5]. Thus, synthetic peptides derived from natural AMPs have been generated. Due to the limitations of natural AMPs, there has been an increasing interest in developing non-peptide analogs that mimic the properties and functions of natural AMPs in order to overcome these limitations [27]. An example of non-peptides AMP mimics are peptide analogs, which are usually developed on small abiotic scaffolds [28]. Early approaches focused on optimizing their microbicidal properties, although often this led to increased levels of cytotoxicity as their natural counterparts. Thus, more recent approaches have focused on mimicking the immunomodulatory properties of AMPs along with their potential microbicidal activity [5, 29].

Exogenous administration of many AMPs has been found to be effective in various animal models for bacterial, viral, and fungal infections. However, this efficacy can be due in part to immunomodulatory effects and not only direct antimicrobial activity [5]. Studies have shown the potential immunodulatory role of AMPs to treat non-infectious inflammatory diseases such as in arthritis [30], asthma [31], colitis [32], and even cancer [33]. Alternatively, instead of exogenous administration, others had opted for enhancing the expression of endogenous AMPs for chronic inflammatory and infectious disease [5].

Most AMPs and AMPs analogs have reached clinical trial that has been formulated for topical application or as inhalants [34]. However, there are also clinical trials for oral and intravenous AMP or AMP analogs [5]. Some of these clinical trials have reached phase III, despite their development had been terminated [5, 34]. This step missing for full approval to be released in the market has to do with regulations that require new antimicrobial to perform better in terms of efficacy to control infections than existing antibiotics, even if the new compound does not generate antimicrobial resistance [5].

Still, the challenges to bring peptide-based AMP compounds to the market involved formulation, delivery, and costs. Biologically, factors to be considered include peptide stability and bioavailability since pH or proteases present in the body can degrade such peptides. Moreover, other factors present in the host-like physiological salt concentrations, mucus, DNA, and microbial saccharides can impair peptide activity [5].

This book will be touching a wide variety of aspects in the field of AMPs, from their basic biological roles to their potential use in medicine. The research on AMPs is a growing field that keeps expanding year after year. We expect the reader to use this book as a nutritive source of information to better understand about the field of AMPs and also to encouraging going beyond of what has been embodied here.

Author details

Jorge Masso-Silva[1], Anna Savitskaya[2] and Shymaa Enany[3*]

1 Division of Pulmonary Critical Care and Sleep, Section Chief of Pulmonary Critical Care Medicine, University of California at San Diego, San Diego, USA

2 Institute of Bioorganic Chemistry of Russian Academy of Science, Moscow, Russian Federation

3 Microbiology and Immunology Department, Faculty of Pharmacy, Suez Canal University, Egypt

*Address all correspondence to: shymaa21@yahoo.com

References

[1] Hancock REW, Diamond G. The role of cationic antimicrobial peptides in innate host defences. Trends in Microbiology. 2000;**8**:402-410

[2] Hancock RE, Haney EF, Gill EE. The immunology of host defence peptides: Beyond antimicrobial activity. Nature Reviews. Immunology. 2016;**16**:321-334

[3] Kumar P, Kizhakkedathu JN, Straus SK. Antimicrobial peptides: Diversity, mechanism of action and strategies to improve the activity and biocompatibility in vivo. Biomolecules. 2018;**8**(1):4

[4] Shafee TM, Lay FT, Phan TK, Anderson MA, Hulett MD. Convergent evolution of defensin sequence, structure and function. Cellular and Molecular Life Sciences. 2017;**74**: 663-682

[5] Mookherjee N, Anderson MA, Haagsman HP, Davidson DJ. Antimicrobial host defence peptides: Functions and clinical potential. Nature Reviews Drug Discovery. 2020;**19**: 311-332

[6] Steiner H, Hultmark D, Engström Å, Bennich H, Boman HG. Sequence and specificity of two antibacterial proteins involved in insect immunity. Nature. 1981;**292**:246-248

[7] Masso-Silva JA, Diamond G. Antimicrobial peptides from fish. Pharmaceuticals (Basel). 2014;**7**:265-310

[8] Wang G, Li X, Wang Z. APD3: The antimicrobial peptide database as a tool for research and education. Nucleic Acids Research. 2016;**44**:D1087-D1093

[9] Parisi K, Shafee TMA, Quimbar P, van der Weerden NL, Bleackley MR, Anderson MA. The evolution, function and mechanisms of action for plant defensins. Seminars in Cell & Developmental Biology. 2019;**88**:107-118

[10] Huan Y, Kong Q, Mou H, Yi H. Antimicrobial peptides: Classification, design, application and research progress in multiple fields. Frontiers in Microbiology. 2020;**11**:582779. DOI: 10.3389/fmicb.2020.582779

[11] Yang D, Biragyn A, Hoover DM, Lubkowski J, Oppenheim JJ. Multiple roles of antimicrobial defensins, cathelicidins, and eosinophil-derived Neurotoxin in host defense. Annual Review of Immunology. 2004;**22**:181-215

[12] Menzel LP, Chowdhury HM, Masso-Silva JA, et al. Potent in vitro and in vivo antifungal activity of a small molecule host defense peptide mimic through a membrane-active mechanism. Scientific Reports. 2017;**7**:4353

[13] Ryan LK, Freeman KB, Masso-Silva JA, et al. Activity of potent and selective host defense peptide mimetics in mouse models of oral candidiasis. Antimicrobial Agents and Chemotherapy. 2014;**58**:3820-3827

[14] Oshiro KGN, Rodrigues G, Monges BED, Cardoso MH, Franco OL. Bioactive peptides against fungal biofilms. Frontiers in Microbiology. 2019;**10**:2169. DOI: 10.3389/fmicb.2019.02169

[15] van der Does AM, Hiemstra PS, Mookherjee N. Antimicrobial host defence peptides: Immunomodulatory functions and translational prospects. Advances in Experimental Medicine and Biology. 2019;**1117**:149-171

[16] Dadgostar P. Antimicrobial resistance: implications and costs. Infection and Drug Resistance. 2019;**12**:3903-3910

[17] Friedman ND, Temkin E, Carmeli Y. The negative impact of antibiotic resistance. Clinical Microbiology and Infection. 2016;**22**:416-422

[18] Wiederhold NP. Antifungal resistance: Current trends and future

strategies to combat. Infection and Drug Resistance. 2017;**10**:249-259

[19] Fernández de Ullivarri M, Arbulu S, Garcia-Gutierrez E, Cotter PD. Antifungal peptides as therapeutic agents. Frontiers in Cellular and Infection Microbiology. 2020;**10**:105. doi: 10.3389/fcimb.2020.00105

[20] Ahmed A, Siman-Tov G, Hall G, Bhalla N, Narayanan A. Human antimicrobial peptides as therapeutics for viral infections. Viruses. 2019;**11**(8):704. DOI: 10.3390/v11080704

[21] Vizioli J, Salzet M. Antimicrobial peptides versus parasitic infections? Trends in Parasitology. 2002;**18**:475-476

[22] Andersson DI, Hughes D, Kubicek-Sutherland JZ. Mechanisms and consequences of bacterial resistance to antimicrobial peptides. Drug Resistance Updates. 2016;**26**:43-57

[23] Joo HS, Fu CI, Otto M. Bacterial strategies of resistance to antimicrobial peptides. Philosophical Transactions of the Royal Society of London. Series B, Biological Sciences. 2016;**371**(1695): 20150292

[24] Sahl HG, Shai Y. Bacterial resistance to antimicrobial peptides. Biochimica et Biophysica Acta. 2015; **1848**:3019-3020

[25] El Shazely B, Urbański A, Johnston PR, Rolff J. In vivo exposure of insect AMP resistant Staphylococcus aureus to an insect immune system. Insect Biochemistry and Molecular Biology. 2019;**110**:60-68

[26] Duong L, Gross SP, Siryaporn A. Developing antimicrobial synergy with AMPs. Frontiers in Medical Technology. 2021;**3**:640981. DOI: 10.3389/fmedt.2021.640981

[27] Scott RW, Tew GN. Mimics of host defense proteins; Strategies for translation to therapeutic applications. Current Topics in Medicinal Chemistry. 2017;**17**:576-589

[28] Rotem S, Mor A. Antimicrobial peptide mimics for improved therapeutic properties. Biochimica et Biophysica Acta (BBA) - Biomembranes. 2009;**1788**:1582-1592

[29] Haney EF, Mansour SC, Hilchie AL, de la Fuente-Núñez C, Hancock RE. High throughput screening methods for assessing antibiofilm and immunomodulatory activities of synthetic peptides. Peptides. 2015;**71**:276-285

[30] Chow LN, Choi KY, Piyadasa H, et al. Human cathelicidin LL-37-derived peptide IG-19 confers protection in a murine model of collagen-induced arthritis. Molecular Immunology. 2014;**57**:86-92

[31] Piyadasa H, Hemshekhar M, Altieri A, et al. Immunomodulatory innate defence regulator (IDR) peptide alleviates airway inflammation and hyper-responsiveness. Thorax. 2018;**73**:908-917

[32] Ho S, Pothoulakis C, Koon HW. Antimicrobial peptides and colitis. Current Pharmaceutical Design. 2013;**19**:40-47

[33] Tornesello AL, Borrelli A, Buonaguro L, Buonaguro FM, Tornesello ML. Antimicrobial peptides as anticancer agents: Functional properties and biological activities. Molecules. 19, 2020;**25**(12):2850. DOI: 10.3390/molecules25122850.

[34] Greber KE, Dawgul M. Antimicrobial peptides under clinical trials. Current Topics in Medicinal Chemistry. 2017;**17**:620-628

Chapter 2

Anti-Microbial Peptides: The Importance of Structure-Function Analysis in the Design of New AMPs

Awatef Ouertani, Amor Mosbah and Ameur Cherif

Abstract

In recent years the rapid emergence of drug resistant microorganisms has become a major health problem worldwide. The number of multidrug resistant (MDR) bacteria is in a rapid increase. Therefore, there is an urgent need to develop new antimicrobial agent that is active against MDR. Among the possible candidates, antimicrobial peptides (AMPs) represent a promising alternative. Many AMPs candidates were in clinical development and the Nisin was approved in many food products. Exact mechanism of AMPs action has not been fully elucidated. More comprehensive of the mechanism of action provide a path towards overcoming the toxicity limitation. This chapter is a review that provides an overview of bacterial AMPs named bacteriocin, focusing on their diverse mechanism of action. We develop here the structure–function relationship of many AMPs. A good understanding of AMPS structure–function relationship can helps the scientific in the conception of new active AMPs by the evaluation of the role of each residue and the determination of the essential amino acids for activity. This feature helps the development of the second-generation AMPs with high potential antimicrobial activity and more.

Keywords: Multidrug resistant bacteria, Antimicrobial peptide, mechanism of action, peptide synthesis

1. Introduction

The routinely use of antibiotics decreased their efficiency and allowed bacteria to adapt to antibiotics, resulting in the emergence and rapid propagation of resistant bacterial strain [1]. This feature is a serious health and economic problem, leading to increased rates of morbidity and mortality associated with bacterial infections caused by multi resistant bacteria [2] such as Methicillin-Resistant *Staphylococcus aureus* (MRSA), Vancomycin-Resistant Enterococci (VRE) or MDR [3–5]. To fight against this health problem, it is imperative to find new alternatives to antibiotics [6]. Several resources were investigated, for their ability to provide antimicrobial agent as well as animals, plants derived compounds and microorganisms [7]. Among natural resources, bacteria are known to be a good producer of antimicrobial agents [8] such as lipopeptides, glycopeptides cyclic peptides and natural peptides named as bacteriocins [9–11]. The latter are considered as the first line defense of bacteria and allows them to gain a competitive advantage and to thrive in complex ecosystems [11]. Bacteriocins received a great interest as potential antimicrobial agents with high activity against numerous bacterial, fungal, yeast and viral species [12–14]. Riley et al. have reported that all bacteria are able to produce bacteriocins [15]. A large variety of bacteriocins have been identified, and some bacteria can produce bacteriocins with activity against MDR bacteria [16]. This broad collection of antimicrobial molecules allows many biotechnological, industrial and pharmaceutical applications [17]. Moreover, their toxicity is a limiting factor. Nisin is the only bacteriocin that have been legally approved by the world health organization (WHO) and by the food and drug administration (FDA) for human use as a food preservative, and it has been given a generally-regarded-as-safe (GRAS) designation by the FDA [17]. It is safe for human consumption and is not toxic to animals. Thus, toxicology studies have demonstrated that nisin ingestion does not cause toxic effects to the human body, and LD50 reported was 6950 mg/kg when administered orally [18]. Nisin was shown to be effective against various Gram positive bacteria such as *Listeria monocytogenes, Staphylococcus* aureus, *Bacillus cereus, Bacillus subtilis, Enterococcus faecalis* [19]. In adition, Nisin derivatives are more active [17].

Bacteriocins possess a key treats that makes them a good alternative to antibiotics [20]:

i. They are abundant with large diversity [20, 21].

ii. Various bacteriocins such as nisin [22] have demonstrated distinct mode of action compared to conventional antibiotics.

iii. The use of bacteriocin with narrow spectrum of inhibition preserves the natural healthy microbiota [23].

iv. The long term bacteriocin exposure is safe with no side effects and do not lead to bacterial resistance [24, 25].

The study of bacteriocin structures and amino acids composition helps to understand their detailed mechanism of action. This feature is critical towards the development of bacteriocins as therapeutics and can also be used to prioritize hits in their genome mining studies [26]. Hence a library of synthetic bacteriocin variants served as a tool; to recognize key residues responsible for activity and could continue to inspire the development of new therapeutic agents [27].

2. Bacterial antimicrobial peptides bacteriocins

Bacteriocins are ribosomally synthetised peptides produced by Gram positive, Gram negative bacteria and fungi to kill or inhibit significant pathogenic bacteria [28]. Bacteriocin was discovered for the first time by A. Gratia in 1925 when he was involved in the method of searching for approaches to kill bacteria. The first bacteriocin that inhibited *E. coli was* named colicin [29]. This powerful biological arm allows microorganisms to compete for resources and space [11]. Bacteriocin can be incorporated in the food products as purified or semi purified form also the producer strain can incorporated. Nisin is exploited in various commercial preparations, such as Nisaplin, Chrisin and DelvoNis. It is commonly used in dairy industries to control clostridia and post-processing contamination from Listeria strains [30].

Furthermore, nisin and further bacteriocins have been shown to inhibit several pathogens in many food matrixes. Many studies have demonstrated the anti-biofilm properties of nisin and the capacity to act synergistically in combination with conventional therapeutic drugs [31]. In addition, nisin could stimulate the adaptive immune response with an immunomodulatory function. Also, nisin can control the growth of tumors and exhibit selective cytotoxicity towards cancer cells [32]. Bacteriocins have also been identified as promising next generation antibiotics to combat MDR pathogens [33].

2.1 Classification

During the years of discovery, numerous approaches have been taken to classify bacteriocins into a number of groups. This includes the nature of the producing strains, the methods by which these molecules are produced, common resistance mechanisms and the peptides mechanism of actions [34]. The most useful classification established by Claenhamer et al. (1993) subdivides bacteriocin into four classes [35] as follow:

ClassI: small bacteriocin with a molecular weight less than 5 kDa, heat stable and harbor non-standard amino acids such as lanthionine, β methyllanthionine, dehydrobulyrine, dehydroalanine and labyrinthine [36]. Class I is subdivided into:

i. class Ia (lantibiotics): consists of flexible, elongated, positively charged, and hydrophobic peptides associated with a pore formation in bacterial membranes. Nisin is the most representative bacteriocin of this group.

ii. class Ib (labyrinthopeptins): it regroups globular and inflexible bacteriocins that are negatively charged or with no net charge. These bacteriocins can inhibit catalytic enzymes crucial for the proliferation of susceptible bacteria [37].

iii. class Ic (sanctibiotics) are sulfur-to-α-carbon-containing peptides [38]. Nisin is the most studied class I bacteriocin [39].

ClassII: Class II bacteriocin regroups peptides with a molecular weight less than 10 kDa, heat stable and with no modified amino acids. This class is subdivided into four sub-classes. Class IIa also named pediocin like bacteriocins [40]. It regroups bacteriocin typically comprised of 25–28 AA with a conserved amino acid sequence YGNGV on their *N*-terminal domains [41]. Class IIb or two peptides bacteriocin. This class regroups two different peptides, both are essential for the antimicrobial activity [37]. Class IIc: circular bacteriocins produced by Gram-positive bacteria represent a diverse class of antimicrobial peptides that are more stable compared to linear bacteriocins [42]. Class IId: linear non-pediocin-like one-peptide bacteriocins [43].

Class III: the large and heat labile bacteriocins. Colicin is one of the well-characterized Class III bacteriocin They have a bacteriolytic (IIIa) or nonlytic mechanism of action (class IIIb) [44].

Class IV: this class regroups complex protein associated with one or more chemical moieties either lipid or carbohydrate [45].

2.2 Biosynthesis

Bacteriocins are primary metabolites with simpler biosynthetic machinery [46]. Bacteriocin coding genes are generally in operon clusters with the minimum genetic machinery, composed of the structural gene and the associated immunity. The clusters harbored in the genome, plasmid or other mobile genetic elements [47].

Bacteriocins are synthesized as inactive precursor peptides composed of an N-terminal leader peptide close to the C-terminal pro-peptide. The leader peptide serves as a recognition site for the biosynthetic enzymes implicated in the maturation process and its transport outside of the producer strain [2]. Bacteriocins are transported and cleaved to generate the mature form through enzymatic processes [48]. Recently, various leaderless bacteriocin has been reported [49, 50] with no common biosynthesis and regulation mechanism [51]. Leaderless bacteriocins do not undergo post translational modification and become active after [51]. Coelho et al. (2016) have reported that a complex mechanism involving a protein with a helix-turn-helix (HTH) AurR, an alternative transcription factor σ^B, and a phage regulator ϕ11, regulates the production of aureocin A70 [52]. An ABC-type multidrug resistance transporter protein, LmrB, has been reported to be implicated in secretion and immunity of the LsbB, leaderless bacteriocin [53].

2.3 Mode of action

Usually, Gram-negative bacteria are naturally resistant to the bacteriocins, due to their outer membrane, which acts as an effective barrier [54, 55]. Microcin B17 (MccB17) is an antibacterial peptide produced by strains of *Escherichia coli* harboring the plasmid-borne mccB17 operon [56]. This bacteriocin passes through the outer membrane via the porin OmpF and is transferred across the inner membrane in a manner that is dependent on the inner-membrane peptide transporter SbmA. The bacteriocin then acts by inhibiting DNA gyrase-mediated DNA supercoiling, thus interfering with DNA replication [20].

The bacteriocin MccJ25 is recognized by the iron siderophore receptor FhuA at the outer membrane and requires TonB and SbmA at the inner membrane to go through the cell. After entering the cell, MccJ25 block the secondary channel of RNA polymerase resulting on the transcription inhibition [57]. MccC7-C51, passes through the inner layer of the *E. coli* cell wall via the YejABEF transporter [58], after which the bacteriocin is processed by one of the many broad-specificity cytoplasmic aminopeptidases of the bacterium [59] to generate a modified aspartyl-adenylate. This, in turn, inhibits aspartyl-tRNA synthetase, thus blocking mRNA synthesis (**Figure 1**) [20].

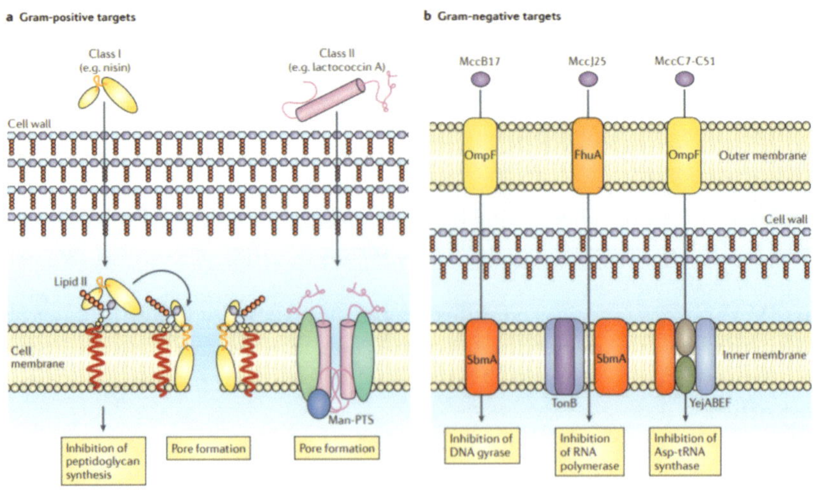

Figure 1.
Illustration of mechanism of action of representative bacteriocins that inhibit gram-positive (a) and gram-negative bacteria [20].

The general cationic nature of bacteriocins plays a key role in their initial interaction with the cell membrane of the target strains. The negative charge of bacterial cell membranes and the positive charge of bacteriocin generate an electrostatic interaction between them, thus facilitating the approach of the molecules to the membranes [60]. Lantibiotic such as nisin have dual killing mechanism that require its interaction with lipid II receptor leading to i) pore forming that induces the dissipation of the membrane potential and the efflux of small metabolites such as ions, amino acids, nucleotides and other cytoplasmic solutes, resulting in the execution of all biosynthetic processes and the cell death. ii) prevention of peptidoglycan, the main component of the bacterial cell wall, synthesis, causing cell death [61]. Whereas, Members of class IIa bacteriocins have been shown to bind to mannose phosphotransferase system (Man-PTS) proteins, the sugar-uptake system of target bacteria, to exhibit their antimicrobial activity [62]. Their anti listerial activity is due to the conserved N-terminal YGNGV motif, while the less conserved C-terminal domain is responsible for their antimicrobial activity against other strains [41]. Circular bacteriocin such as enterocin AS-48, gassericin A, subtilosin A, and carnocyclin do not require a receptor molecule for their activity. Their basic amino acid residues patch on the surface of their compact hydrophobic globular structure was responsible for the electrostatic interaction between the bacteriocin and the surface membrane of the target cell [63]. However, garvicin ML, a new member of circular bacteriocins, exhibits its activity through binding to a maltose ABC-transporter protein as a target receptor of garvicin ML, which facilitates the efflux of intracellular solutes resulting to the cell death [42].

Leaderless bacteriocins have been shown to not involve a receptor molecule to exhibit their antimicrobial activity [51]. Fujita et al. [64] characterized the mode of action of Lacticin Q, leaderless bacteriocins produced by *L. lactis QU* 5. It demonstrates antimicrobial activity against various Gram-positive bacteria such as *Bacillus sp., Lactobacillus sp., Enterococcus sp., Lactococcus sp., and Staphylococcus aureus* [64]. Lacticin Q has been shown to form toroidal pore (HTP) causing depletion of intracellular components such as proteins, ions and ATP, leading to cell death. The HTP formation mechanism initiates with the electrostatic interaction of the cationic lacticin Q and the negatively charged membranes. These binding results in the formation of HTPs associated with lipid flip-flop [51]. In addition, the leaderless aureocin A53 produced by *S. aureus* A53 was shown to permeate the membranes of the bacteria without forming pores [65]. It demonstrates stronger interaction with

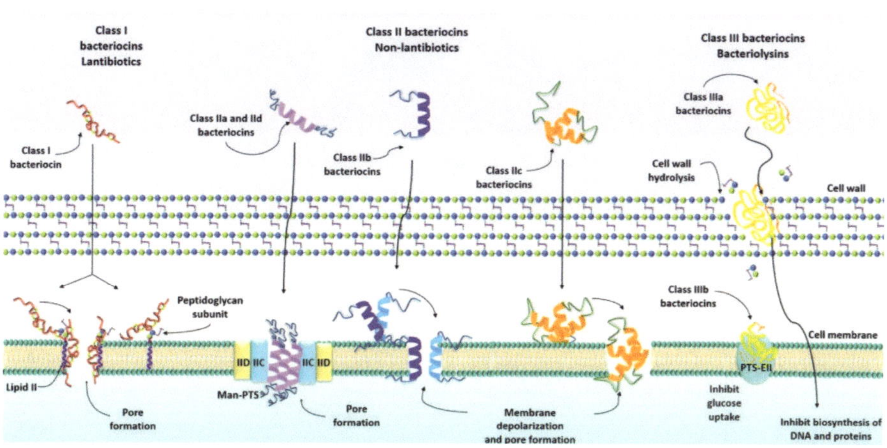

Figure 2.
Illustration of different mechanism of action of three classes' bacteriocins [37].

neutral membrane rather than negatively charged lipids. Studies on the leaderless bacteriocin, LsbB, isolated from *L. lactis subsp. lactis* BGMN1–5, shed light on a zinc-dependent membrane metallopeptidase, YvjB, as its receptor molecule [66]. The C-terminal end of LsbB harbors the receptor binding domain [67] that interacts with the highly conserved Tyr356 and Ala353 residues located at the transmembrane domain of YvjB [68] (**Figures 1** and **2**).

2.4 Structural analysis: amino acids and activity

NMR resolution structure of circular bacteriocins such as; enterocin AS-48, carnocyclin A, enterocin NKR 5-3B and acidocin B demonstrates a conserved structural motif consisting of four to five α-helices surrounding a hydrophobic core, with the C-terminus and N-terminus ligation occurring within an helix secondary structure [63, 69–72] (**Figure 3**). Various studies suggested that the circularization is not essential for antimicrobial activity but more important for stabilization of the three-dimensional structure of the bacteriocin [73–76]. Jimenez et al. (2005) demonstrated that a fragment of enterocin AS-48 harboring the cationic putative membrane interacting region exhibited competitive membrane binding with no antibacterial activity. This result suggests that the cationic surface patches are involved in an initial electrostatic interaction between the peptide and the negatively charged phospholipids bilayer of target cell membrane. Furthermore, other physicochemical properties of the bacteriocins may be required for antimicrobial action [42, 51, 77]. Additionally, mutation of aromatic residues in AS-48 reduced activity which shed light on the role of aromatic amino acids on antimicrobial activity.

Furthermore, the crystal structure and site directed mutagenesis of plantacyclin B21AG reveals that Phe8, Trp45 and Lys19 are essential for antimicrobial activity and a significant reduction in activity was observed with Alanine substitution mutagenesis supporting the notion of a similar role of these residues [78] (**Figure 4**). Moreover, many Trp rich AMPs (TrAMPs) has shown interesting antifungal activity such as synthetic peptides PW2 [79], PAF2 [80] and PEP6 [81]. Also, Blondelle et al. have synthesized Combi-1, Combi-2 and Cyclo-Combi, three TrAMPs with high antimicrobial activity against *E.coli, S.aureus, S.sanguis and C.albicans* [82].

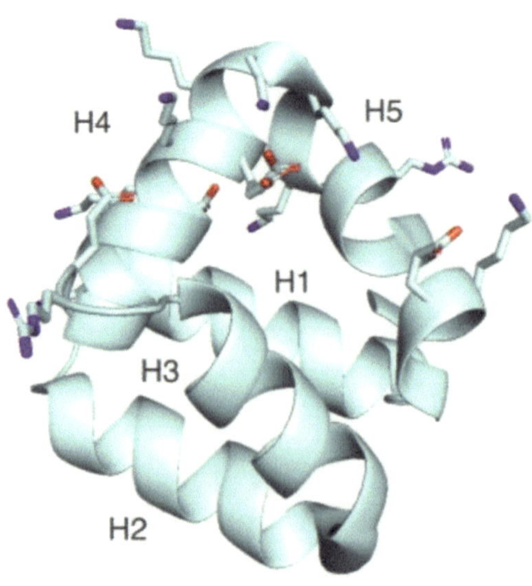

Figure 3.
Crystal structure of AS-48 (PDB 1O82) [26].

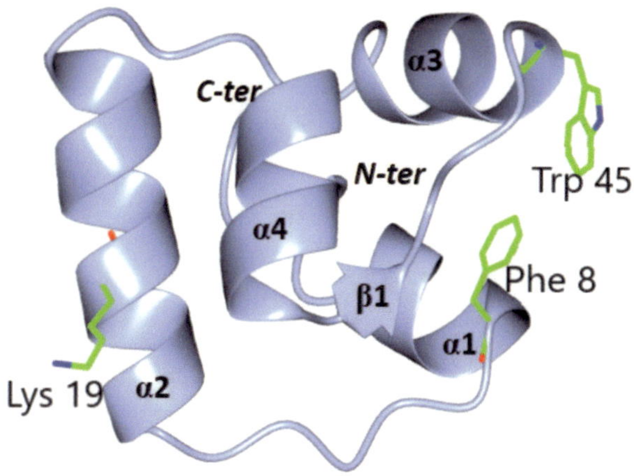

Figure 4.
Crystal structure of B21AG showing amino acids essential for activity [78].

Trp residues are always associated with Arg residues which have a positively charged guanidium group located at the end of the side chain. This group ensures i) the attraction of the TrAMPs to target membranes by forming hydrogen bonds with the negatively charged membrane component. ii) Electrostatic and H-bonding with anionic and polar molecule resulting on the cell penetrating peptides. These distinctive properties are crucial for the highly activity of the Arg and Trp –rich peptides even at very short peptide lengths [83].

Various studies have illuminated the picture of structural and functional relationships in nisin. Thus, the specific mutation shed light on the key regions essential for antimicrobial activity. N-terminal was found to be crucial for nisin binding to the lipidII pyrophosphate region [84]. Therefore, the first two residues IL1 and Dhb2 associated with N-ter lanthhionine ring A and methyl lanthionine ringB forms a pocket that encloses the lipidII. This interaction is ensured by the hydrogen binding between the pyrophosphate group of lipidII and the backbone amides [26]

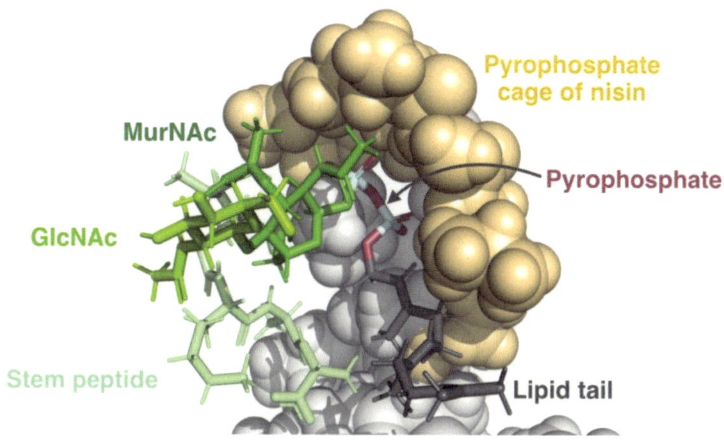

Figure 5.
NMR structure (PDB: 1WCO) of nisin bound to a lipid II analog. Nisin is shown as a space-filling model and the lipid II analog is shown as sticks. The N-terminal (methyl)lanthionine rings (space-filling tan) of nisin envelop the pyrophosphate moiety (magenta and cyan sticks) of lipid II [26].

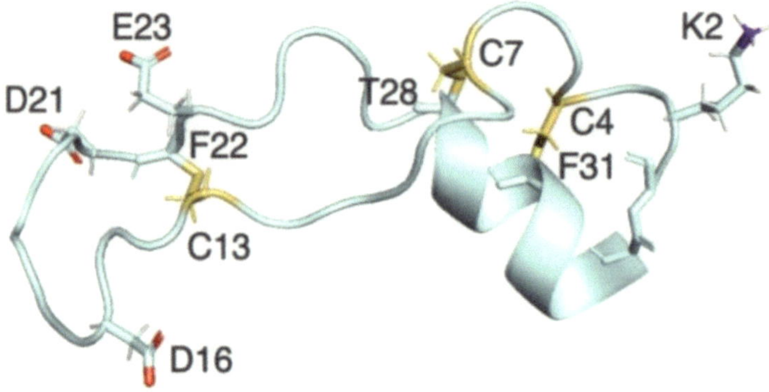

Figure 6.
The crystal structure of subtilosin A (PDB:1PXQ) illustrates a rigid hairpin-like structure. Acidic (D16, D21, E23) and basic (K2) amino acids are localized at different ends of the folded peptide. Residues participating in thioether linkages are shown as gold sticks [26].

(**Figure 5**). Wiedemann et al. have demonstrated that C-terminal region is crucial for binding to membrane with a negative surface charge. However, aa33 and aa34 did not play any role in vivo activity [85]. Also, the substitution of Val32 by Lys or Glu residue results on the drastic decrease of activity associated with a significant reduction on K^+ release. This feature demonstrated that the presence of a charged residue in the central segment of the molecule is not tolerable and affect the pore forming process [85]. The C and N-terminal regions are separated by a few residues that proceed as a flexible pivot around which the C-terminal of nisin can rotate and insert vertically into the phospholipids bilayer [26].

Subtilosin A a bacteriocin produced by *B.subtilis* was also characterized. It is composed of three cyclic segments. The intramolecular linkages are ensured by three thioether bridges connecting C4 with F31, C7 with T28, and C13 with F22, while an amide bond between N1 and G35 links the N- and C-terminus of the peptide (**Figure 6**). This feature contributes to the semi-rigid, cyclic nature of subtilosin A [86–88]. Subtilosin A contain many hydrophobic residues, but there are also three acidic residues, two Aspartate and one glutamate, that are localized on the loop end of the folded peptide and a basic residue,Lysine, present on the opposite end. This separation of charge confers a net anionic (−2). Thus, like bacteriocin, the model proposed for binding engages insertion of the loop-distal end of subtilosin A into the lipid bilayer first [88]. This end harbors the single basic residue, K2, which may interact with the negatively charged phosphate headgroup and a large, hydrophobic tryptophan residue, W34, which may disturb the lipid bilayer [88]. The insertion of subtilosin A causes an ATP efflux and a reduction of the transmembrane ion gradient [89].

3. Conclusion

In recent years, the increased number of MDR pathogens has become a serious problem, and developing a new generation of antimicrobial agents is becoming urgent.

Increased interest has been shown in bacteriocin, AMPs produced by bacteria, particularly the one produced by lactic acid bacteria (LAB) [90]. Numerous bacteriocins have been shown to be effective against many pathogenic bacteria [24]; however, Nisin is the only bacteriocin legally approved by the WHO and by FDA for use in the food, medicine and veterinary industry [91]. Many, derivatives of nisin have been developed and used in various applications.

Bacteriocins are diverse with different mechanism of action. A deepest comprehensive of mechanism of action and the identification of key amino acids and receptor crucial for activity helps to understand the detailed mechanism of action. This feature leads to the development of new antibiotics effective against MDR bacteria and to solve the problem of bacterial resistance.

To address this issue, in this chapter, we have compiled available data to shed light on the structural function relationship of various bacteriocins.

Author details

Awatef Ouertani*, Amor Mosbah and Ameur Cherif
University of Manouba, ISBST, BVBGR-LR11ES31, Biotechpole Sidi Thabet, Ariana, Tunisia

*Address all correspondence to: awatef.ouertani@gmail.com

References

[1] Gould IM (2009). Antibiotic resistance: The perfect storm. Int J Antimicrob Agents 34:S2–S5.

[2] Simons A, Alhanout K, Duval RE (2020). Bacteriocins, Antimicrobial Peptides from Bacterial Origin: Overview of Their Biology and Their Impact against Multidrug-Resistant Bacteria. Microorganisms 8(5):639.

[3] Xia J, Gao J, Kokudo N, Hasegawa K, Tang W (2013). Methicillin-resistant *Staphylococcus aureus* antibiotic resistance and virulence. Biosci. Trends 7:113-121.

[4] Giamarellou H, Poulakou G (2009). Multidrug-Resistant Gram-Negative Infections. Drugs 69:1879-1901.

[5] Calfee DP (2012). Methicillin-resistant *Staphylococcus aureus* and vancomycin-resistant enterococci, and other Gram-positives in healthcare. Curr Opin Infect Dis 25:385.

[6] Duval RE, Grare M, Demoré B (2019). Fight Against Antimicrobial Resistance: We Always Need New Antibacterials but for Right Bacteria. Molecules. 24(17):3152.

[7] Mbaveng AT, Sandjo LP, Tankeo SB, Ndifor AR, Pantaleon A, Nagdjui BT, Kuete V (2015). Antibacterial activity of nineteen selected natural products against multi-drug resistant Gram-negative phenotypes Springer plus 30 (4):823.

[8] Abriouel H, Franz CM, Ben Omar N, Galvez A (2011). Diversity and application of Bacillus bacteriocins. FEMS Microbiol Rev 35:201-232.

[9] Kleinkauf H, von Döhren H. Review Nonribosomal biosynthesis of peptide antibiotics. In: Christen P, Hofmann E, editors. EJB Reviews 1990. Springer; Berlin/Heidelberg, Germany: 1991. pp. 151-165. European Journal of Biochemistry

[10] Saadouli I, Zendah El Euch I, Trabelsi E, Mosbah A, Redissi A, Ferjani R, Fhoula I, Cherif A, Sabatier JM, Sewald N, Ouzari HI (2020). Isolation, Characterization and Chemical Synthesis of Large Spectrum Antimicrobial Cyclic Dipeptide (l-leu-l-pro) from *Streptomyces misionensis* V16R3Y1 Bacteria Extracts. A Novel ^{1}H NMR Metabolomic Approach. Antibiotics (Basel). 21;9(5):270.

[11] Ouertani A, Chaabouni I, Mosbah A, Long J, Barakat M, Mansuelle P, Mghirbi O, Najjari A, Ouzari H-I, Masmoudi AS, Maresca M, Ortet P, Gigmes D, Mabrouk K and Cherif A (2018) Two New Secreted Proteases Generate a Casein-Derived Antimicrobial Peptide in *Bacillus cereus* Food Born Isolate Leading to Bacterial Competition in Milk Front. Microbiol. 9:1148.

[12] Chi H, Holo H (2018). Synergistic Antimicrobial Activity Between the Broad Spectrum Bacteriocin Garvicin KS and Nisin, Farnesol and Polymyxin B Against Gram-Positive and Gram-Negative Bacteria Curr Microbiol 75(3):272-277.

[13] Smaoui S, Elleuch L, Bejar W, Karray-Rebai I, Ayadi I, Jaouadi B, Mathieu F, Chouayekh H, Bejar S, Mellouli L (2010). Inhibition of fungi and gram-negative bacteria by bacteriocin BacTN635 produced by *Lactobacillus plantarum* sp. TN635 Appl Biochem Biotechnol 162(4):1132-1146

[14] Sharma A, Srivastava S (2014). Anti-Candida activity of two-peptide bacteriocins, plantaricins (Pln E/F and J/K) and their mode of action Fungal Biol 118(2):264-275.

[15] Riley M A, Wertz J E (2002). Bacteriocins: evolution, ecology, and

application. Annu Rev Microbiol 56: 117-137 .

[16] El-Gendy, A.O., Brede, D.A., Essam, T.M. et al (2021). Purification and characterization of bacteriocins-like inhibitory substances from food isolated Enterococcus faecalis OS13 with activity against nosocomial enterococci Sci Rep 11, 3795.

[17] Kamarajan P, Hayami T, Matte B, Liu Y, Danciu T, Ramamoorthy A, et al. (2015). Nisin ZP, a Bacteriocin and Food Preservative, Inhibits Head and Neck Cancer Tumorigenesis and Prolongs Survival. PLoS ONE 10(7): e0131008.

[18] Jozala AF, Novaes L.CdL, Júnior AP. (Nisin 2015). In Concepts, Compounds and the Alternatives of Antibacterials IntechOpen: London, UK: 103-119.

[19] Sukrita PP, Parichat P, Pongsak R 2015. Nisin: production and mechanism of antimicrobial action. Int J Cur Res Rev 7 (2): 47-53.

[20] Cotter PD, Ross RP, Hill C (2013). Bacteriocins - a viable alternative to antibiotics? Nat Rev Microbiol 11(2):95-105.

[21] Yang SC, Lin CH, Sung CT, Fang JY (2014). Antibacterial activities of bacteriocins: application in foods and pharmaceuticals Front Microbiol 26(5):241.

[22] Campion A, Casey PG, Field D et al (2013). In vivo activity of Nisin A and Nisin V against Listeria monocytogenes in mice BMC Microbiol 13(23).

[23] Francino MP (2016). Antibiotics and the Human Gut Microbiome: Dysbioses and Accumulation of Resistances Front Microbiol 12(6):1543.

[24] Soltani S, Hammami R, Cotter PD, Rebuffat S, Ben Said L, Gaudreau H, Bédard F, Biron E, Drider D, Fliss I(2021). Bacteriocins as a new generation of antimicrobials: toxicity aspects and regulations. FEMS microbial Rev45(1): fuaa039.

[25] Hagiwara A, Imai N, Nakashima H, Toda Y, Kawabe M, Furukawa F, Delves-Broughton J, Yasuhara K, Hayashi SM (2010). A 90-day oral toxicity study of nisin A, an anti-microbial peptide derived from Lactococcus lactis subsp. lactis, in F344 rats Food Chem Toxicol 48(8-9):2421-2428.

[26] Cao L, Turq D, James Link A (2021). Mechanisms of action of ribosomally synthesized and posttranslationally modified peptides (RiPPs) J Ind Microbiol. Biotechnol 48.

[27] O' Connor PM, O' Shea EF, Cotter PD et al (2018). The potency of the broad spectrum bacteriocin, bactofencin A, against staphylococci is highly dependent on primary structure, N-terminal charge and disulphide formation Sci Rep 8:118-133.

[28] Benítez-Chao DF, León-Buitimea A, Lerma-Escalera JA , Morones-Ramírez JR (2021). Bacteriocins: An Overview of Antimicrobial, Toxicity, and Biosafety Assessment by in vivo Models Front Microbiol 12:630-695.

[29] Gratia A (1925). Sur un remarquable example d'antagonisme entre deux souches de colibacille. Comput Rend Soc Biol 93: 1040-1042.

[30] Thomas LV, Delves-Broughton J (2001). New Advances in the Application of the Food Preservative Nisin Res Adv Food Sci 2: 11-22.

[31] Shin JM, Gwak JW, Kamarajan P, Fenno JC, Rickard AH, Kapila YL (2016). Biomedical applications of nisin. J Appl Microbiol 120(6):1449-1465.

[32] Kaur S, Kaur S (2015). Bacteriocins as Potential Anticancer Agents. Front Pharmacol 6:272.

[33] Perez R H, Zendo T, Sonomoto K (2014). Novel bacteriocins from lactic acid bacteria (LAB): various structures and applications Microb Cell Fact 13 (1) .

[34] Chikindas ML, Weeks R, Drider D, Chistyakov VA, Dicks LM (2018). Functions and emerging applications of bacteriocins Curr Opin Biotechnol 49:23-28.

[35] Klaenhammer TR(1993). Genetics of bacteriocins produced by lactic acid bacteria FEMS Microbiol Rev 12: 39-86.

[36] Parada JL, Caron CR, Medeiros ABP, Soccol CR (2007). Bacteriocins from lactic acid bacteria: purification, properties and use as biopreservatives, Braz Arch Biol Technol 50: 521-525.

[37] Hernández-González JC, Martínez-Tapia A, Lazcano-Hernández G, García-Pérez BE, Castrejón-Jiménez NS (2021). Bacteriocins from Lactic Acid Bacteria. A Powerful Alternative as Antimicrobials, Probiotics, and Immunomodulators in Veterinary Medicine Animals 11: 979.

[38] Alvarez-Sieiro P, Montalbán-López M, Mu D, Kuipers OP (2016). Bacteriocins of Lactic Acid Bacteria: Extending the Family Appl MicrobiolBiotechnol. 100: 2939-2951.

[39] Le Lay C, Dridi L, Bergeron M.G, Ouellette M, Fliss I (2016). Nisin is an effective inhibitor of Clostridium difficile vegetative cells and spore germination. J Med Microbiol 65: 169-175.

[40] Bédard F, Biron E (2018). Recent Progress in the Chemical Synthesis of Class II and S-Glycosylated Bacteriocins Front Microbiol 9, 1048.

[41] Fimland G, Johnsen L, Dalhus B, Nissen-Meyer J (2005). Pediocin-like Antimicrobial Peptides (Class IIa Bacteriocins) and Their Immunity Proteins: Biosynthesis, Structure, and Mode of Action J Pept Sci 11: 688-696.

[42] Gabrielsen C, Brede D A, Nes I F, Diep D B (2014). Circular bacteriocins: biosynthesis and mode of action Appl Environ Microbiol 80: 6854-6862.

[43] Angelopoulou A, Warda AK, O'Connor PM, Stockdale SR, Shkoporov AN, Field D, Draper LA, Stanton C, Hill C and Ross RP (2020). Diverse Bacteriocins Produced by Strains From the Human Milk Microbiota Front Microbiol 11:788.

[44] Sun Z, Wang X, Zhang X, Wu H, Zou Y, Li P, Sun C, Xu W, Liu F, Wang D. Class III bacteriocin Helveticin-M causes sublethal damage on target cells through impairment of cell wall and membrane (2018) J Ind Microbiol Biotechnol 45(3):213-227.

[45] Mduduzi Paul Mokoena (2017). Lactic Acid Bacteria and Their Bacteriocins: Classification, Biosynthesis and Applications against Uropathogens: A Mini-Review Molecules 22(8): 1255.

[46] Pham JV, Yilma MA, Feliz A, Majid MT, Maffetone N, Walker JR, Kim E, Cho HJ, Reynolds JM, Song MC, Park SR and Yoon YJ (2019) A Review of the Microbial Production of Bioactive Natural Products and Biologics Front Microbiol 10:1404.

[47] Azevedo AC, Bento CB, Ruiz JC, Queiroz MV, Mantovani HC (2015). Distribution and Genetic Diversity of Bacteriocin Gene Clusters in Rumen Microbial Genomes Appl Environ Microbiol 81(20):7290-7304.

[48] Todorov SD (2009). Bacteriocins from *Lactobacillus plantarum* - production, genetic organization and mode of action: produção, organização genética e modo de ação Braz J Microbiol 40(2):209-221.

[49] Iwatani S, Zendo T, Sonomoto K (2011). Class IId or Linear and Non-Pediocin-Like Bacteriocins Prokaryotic Antimicrob Peptides 237-252

[50] Masuda Y et al (2011). Identifcation and characterization of leucocyclicin Q, a novel cyclic bacteriocin produced by *Leuconostoc mesenteroides* TK41401 Appl Environ Microbiol 77: 8164-8170.

[51] Perez RH, Zendo T , Sonomoto K (2018). Circular and Leaderless Bacteriocins: Biosynthesis, Mode of Action, Applications, and Prospects. Front Microbiol 9:2085.

[52] Coelho ML, Fleming LR, Bastos Mdo C(2016). Insights into aureocin A70 regulation: participation of regulator AurR, alternative transcription factor σ(B) and phage ϕ11 regulator cI Res Microbiol 167(2):90-102.

[53] Gajic O, Buist G, Kojic M, Topisirovic L, Kuipers OP, Kok J. (2003). Novel mechanism of bacteriocin secretion and immunity carried out by lactococcal multidrug resistance proteins J Biol Chem 278: 34291-34298.

[54] Prudêncio CV, Dos Santos MT, Vanetti MC(2015). Strategies for the use of bacteriocins in Gram-negative bacteria: relevance in food microbiology J Food Sci Technol 52(9):5408-5417.

[55] Gyawali R, Ibrahim SA. Natural products as antimicrobial agents. Food Control. 2014;46:412-429. doi: 10.1016/j.foodcont.2014.05.047

[56] Collin f, Maxwell A (2019). The Microbial Toxin Microcin B17: Prospects for the Development of New Antibacterial Agents J Mol Biol 431(18):3400-3426.

[57] Vincent P A, Morero RD (2009). The structure and biological aspects of peptide antibiotic microcin J25, Curr. Med. Chem. 16: 538-549.

[58] Novikova M. et al (2007). The Escherichia coli Yej transporter is required for the uptake of translation inhibitor microcin C. J. Bacteriol 189:8361-8365.

[59] Kazakov T et al (2008). Escherichia coli peptidase A, B, or N can process translation inhibitor microcin C J Bacteriol 190: 2607-2610.

[60] Rodney H. Perez, Maria Teresa M P, Francisco B E (2015). Bacteriocins from Lactic Acid Bacteria: A Review of Biosynthesis, Mode of Action, Fermentative Production, Uses, and Prospects Phil Sci Tech 08(2): 61.

[61] McAuliffe RO, Ross P, Hill C, Lantibiotics: structure, biosynthesis and mode of action (2001), FEMS Microbiology Reviews 25 (3): 285-308.

[62] Tymoszewska A, Diep DB, Wirtek P et al (2017). The Non-Lantibiotic Bacteriocin Garvicin Q Targets Man-PTS in a Broad Spectrum of Sensitive Bacterial Genera Sci Rep 7: 8359.

[63] Van Belkum M J, Martin-Visscher L A Vederas J C(2011). Structure and genetics of circular bacteriocins. Trends Microbiol 19:411-418 .

[64] Fujita K, IchimasaS, Zendo T, Koga S, Yoneyama F, Nakayama J et al (2007). Structural analysis and characterization of lacticin Q, a novel bacteriocin belonging to a new family of unmodified bacteriocins of Grampositive bacteria Appl Environ Microbiol 73: 2871-2877.

[65] Netz D J A, Bastos M, do C, de F, Sahl H G (2002). Mode of action of the antimicrobial peptide aureocin A53 from *Staphylococcus aureus* Appl Environ Microbiol 68: 5274-5280.

[66] Uzelac G, Kojic M, Lozo J, Aleksandrzak-Piekarczyk T, Gabrielsen C, Kristensen T et al. (2013). A Zn-Dependent metallopeptidase is

responsible for sensitivity to LsbB, a class ii leaderless bacteriocin of *Lactococcus lactissubsp*. lactis BGMN1-5 J Bacteriol195: 5614-5621

[67] Ovchinnikov K V, Kristiansen P E, Uzelac G, Topisirovic L, Kojic M, NissenMeyer J et al (2014). Defining the structure and receptor binding domain of the leaderless bacteriocin LsbB J BiolChem 289: 23838-23845.

[68] Miljkovic M, Uzelac G, Mirkovic N, Devescovi G, Diep D B, Venturi V et al. (2016). LsbB bacteriocin interacts with the third transmembrane domain of the YvjB receptor Appl Environ Microbiol 82: 5364-5374.

[69] Himeno K et al (2015). Identifcation, characterization, and three-dimensional structure of the novel circular bacteriocin, enterocin NKR-5-3B, from *Enterococcus faecium* Biochemistry 54:4863-4876 .

[70] Acedo J Z et al (2015). Solution structure of acidocin B, a circular bacteriocin produced by *Lactobacillus acidophilus* M46 Appl Environ Microbiol 81:2910-2918.

[71] Sánchez-Barrena MJ, Martínez-Ripoll M, Gálvez A, et al (2003). Structure of bacteriocin AS-48: From soluble state to membrane bound state J Mol Biol 334:541-549.

[72] Martin-Visscher L A, Gong X, Duszyk M, Vederas J C (2009). Te three-dimensional structure of carnocyclin A reveals that many circular bacteriocins share a common structural motif J Biol Chem 284: 28674-28681.

[73] Montalbán-López M et al (2008). Characterization of linear forms of the circular enterocin AS-48 obtained by limited proteolysis FEBS Lett 582: 3237-3242 .

[74] Sánchez-Hidalgo M et al (2011). AS-48 bacteriocin: close to perfection. Cell Mol Life Sci 68: 2845-2857.

[75] Cobos E et al (2001). AS-48: a circular protein with an extremely stable globular structure. FEBS Lett 505: 379-382 .

[76] Cobos E S et al (2002). The denaturation of circular enterocin AS-48 by urea and guanidinium hydrochloride Biochim Biophys Acta Proteins Proteom 1598: 98-107 .

[77] Jiménez M A, Barrachi-Saccilotto A C, Valdivia E, Maqueda M, Rico M (2004). Design, NMR characterization and activity of a 21-residue peptide fragment of bacteriocin AS-48 containing its putative membrane interacting region J of Pep Sci 11(1): 29-36.

[78] Gor MC, Vezina B, McMahon RM et al (2020). Crystal structure and site-directed mutagenesis of circular bacteriocin plantacyclin B21AG reveals cationic and aromatic residues important for antimicrobial activity Sci Rep 10: 173-98.

[79] Da Silva A, Kawazoe U, Freitas FFT, Gatti MSV, Dolder H, Schumacher RI, Juliano MA, da Silva MJ, Leite A, Avian (2002). Anticoccidial activity of a novel membrane-interactive peptide selected from phage display libraries Mol Biochem Parasitol 120: 53-60.

[80] López-García B Pérez-Payá E Marcos JF (2002). Identification of novel hexapeptides bioactive against phytopathogenic fungi through screening of a synthetic peptide combinatorial library Appl Environ Microbiol 68: 2453-2460.

[81] Reed JD, Edwards DL, Gonzalez CF (1997). Synthetic peptide combinatorial libraries: A method for the identification of bioactive peptides against phytopathogenic fungiMolPlant-Microbe Interact 10: 537-549.

[82] Blondelle SE, Pérez-Payá E, Houghten RA (1996). Synthetic

combinatorial libraries: Novel discovery strategy for identification of antimicrobial agents Antimicrob Agents Chemother 40: 1067-1071.

[83] Awdhesh KM, Jaehyuk C, Eunpyo M, Kwang H B (2018). Tryptophan and Proline rich antimicrobial peptides Molecules 23:815.

[84] Hsu STD, Breukink E, Tischenko E, et al (2004). The nisin-lipid II complex reveals a pyrophosphate cage that provides a blueprint for novel antibiotics Nat Struct Mol Biol 11:963-967.

[85] Wiedemann I, Breukink E, van Kraaij C, Kuipers OP, Bierbaum G, de Kruijff B, SahlHG. (2001). Specific binding of nisin to the peptidoglycan precursor lipid II combines pore formation and inhibition of cell wall biosynthesis for potent antibiotic activity J Biol Chem 276: 1772-1779.

[86] Marx R, Stein T, Entian KD, Glaser SJ (2001). Structure of the Bacillus subtilis peptide antibiotic subtilosin A determined by 1H-NMR and matrix assisted laser desorption/ionization time-of-flight mass spectrometry J Protein Chem 20:501-506.

[87] Kawulka KE, Sprules T, Diaper CM, et al (2004). Structure of Subtilosin A, A Cyclic Antimicrobial Peptide from *Bacillus subtilis* with Unusual Sulfur to α-Carbon Cross-Links: Formation and Reduction of α-Thio-α-Amino Acid Derivatives. Biochemistry 43:3385– 3395.

[88] Thennarasu S, Lee DK, Poon A, Kawulka KE, Vederas JC, Ramamoorthy A. (2005). Membrane permeabilization, orientation, and antimicrobial mechanism of subtilosin A Chem Phys Lipids 137(1-2): 38-51.

[89] Noll KS, Sinko PJ, Chikindas ML, et al (2011). Elucidation of the Molecular Mechanisms of Action of the Natural Antimicrobial Peptide Subtilosin Against the Bacterial Vaginosis associated Pathogen *Gardnerella vaginalis* Probiotics Antimicro 3:41-47.

[90] Vieco-Saiz N, Belguesmia Y, Raspoet R, Auclair E, Gancel F, Kempf I and Drider D (2019). Benefits and Inputs From Lactic Acid Bacteria and Their Bacteriocins as Alternatives to Antibiotic Growth Promoters During Food-Animal Production Front Microbiol 10:57.

[91] Khan I, Oh DH (2016). Integration of nisin into nanoparticles for application in foods Innov Food Sci Emerg Technol 34: 376-384.

Chapter 3

Antimicrobial Peptides: Mechanism of Action

Tanu Singh, Princy Choudhary and Sangeeta Singh

Abstract

Antimicrobial peptides (AMPs) are a diverse class of small peptides that are found in most life forms ranging from microorganisms to humans. They can provoke innate immunity response and show activity against a wide range of microbial cells which includes bacteria, fungi, viruses, parasites, and even cancer cells. In recent years AMPs have gained considerable attention as a therapeutic agent since bacterial resistance towards conventional antibiotics is accelerating rapidly. Thus, it is essential to analyze the mechanism of action (MOA) of AMPs to enhance their use as therapeutics. The MOA of AMPs is classified into two broad categories: direct killing and immunological regulation. The direct killing action mechanism is categorized into membrane targeting and non-membrane targeting mechanisms. There are several models and biophysical techniques which determine the action mechanism of antimicrobial peptides.

Keywords: Antimicrobial peptides, mechanism of action, microbes, membrane disruption, antibiotics

1. Introduction

Antimicrobial peptides (AMPs) are a broad class of small peptide molecules that are found in most life forms ranging from microorganisms to humans. They can provoke an innate immune response in various species, thus they represent the first line of defense against foreign microbes [1]. They show antimicrobial activity against a wide range of microbial cells including bacteria, viruses, fungus, parasites, and even cancer cells. Although, Gram-negative bacteria and Gram-positive bacteria are the most studied targets of AMPs [2]. In recent years AMPs have gained significant attention as potential therapeutic agents since bacterial resistance towards conventional antibiotics is accelerating rapidly [3].

Antimicrobial peptides (AMPs) are considered as attractive alternative antimicrobial agents, as these small biological molecules have mechanism-of-action (MOA) different from the conventional antibiotics, thus they can be applied to combat against various microorganisms even drug-resistant ones [4]. Several properties of these peptides like net charge, hydrophobicity, secondary structure, etc. lead them to have therapeutic action. AMPs are positively charged amphipathic molecules that kill bacteria by using two major MOAs. In the first MOA, AMPs cause membrane disruption, leading to cell lysis and finally cell death. In the second mechanism, AMPs traverse through the cell membrane without disrupting it and inhibit critical intracellular functions by binding to DNA, RNA, or intracellular proteins [5–7]. There are several models which have been used to explain the membrane binding activity of AMPs. Based on the ability to form pores the models are divided into two groups: pore-forming models and non-pore forming models [6]. A large number of biophysical techniques are available that describe their action mechanism whether these peptides disrupt microbial membrane or they target intracellular activities [7].

2. Mechanism of action

AMPs are considered as promising antimicrobial agents due to which their mechanism of action has been explored widely. Characterization of AMPs is very crucial to enhance their utilization as therapeutic agents [6]. Antimicrobial peptides exert both bacteriostatic and bactericidal effects and they develop less resistance to microbes than conventional antibiotics [8].

These peptides are positively charged amphiphilic molecules possessing both hydrophilic and hydrophobic residues. Cationic peptides being positively charged interact with negatively charged cell membranes through electrostatic attraction then undergo membrane adsorption and conformational change. These peptides complete their activity after binding to the cell membrane through different mechanisms such as the barrel stave model, the carpet model, the toroidal pore model, etc. [4]. The mechanisms of action of AMPs differ from antibiotics. There are several hypothetical mechanisms of action of these peptides, including the plasma membrane disruption, intracellular antimicrobial mechanism, the inhibition of the synthesis of macromolecules such as protein, nucleic acids, and enzyme activity, and antimicrobial effect via participating in immune regulatory effects [9, 10].

AMPs are divided into four major types based on their secondary structure including linear α-helical peptides, β-sheet peptides, linear extended peptides, and both α-helix and β-sheet peptides [11]. According to extensive research on members of all four groups of AMPs, the permeabilization of microbial cytoplasmic membranes appears to be the main mechanism for most AMPs to kill cells [2]. The helical peptides damage membranes through the carpet or barrel-stave pore model. Their main function is to introduce amphipathic helices into bacterial cell membranes, which disrupts the structure of the membranes [12]. The β-sheet peptides can act in a variety of ways, including prevention of cell wall formation and binding to particular lipid components in membranes [2]. They translocate across lipid bilayers which are associated with the development of temporary pores. The αβ family contains both α and β structures. Elongated AMPs are linear and rich in one or more amino acids, like glycine, tryptophan, arginine, and histidine. The members of this category have a flexible structure in the aqueous environment that allows them to convert into an amphipathic structure when they come into contact with a membrane. They do not act directly on pathogen membranes, but rather permeate them and interact with cytoplasmic proteins.

The MOA of AMPs can be broadly classified into two categories –first is direct killing and second is immunological regulation as shown in **Figure 1**. The direct killing MOA is further classified into two classes – membrane targeting and non-membrane targeting. Membrane permeabilizing peptides are capable to create transient pores on the membrane, mostly recognized by cationic peptides, such as defensin, LL37, melittin. Non-membrane targeting peptides can pass through the cell membrane and interfere with crucial cellular processes that ultimately lead to the death of cells without permeabilizing the membrane such as pleurocidin, pyrrhocidin, and mersacidin [9].

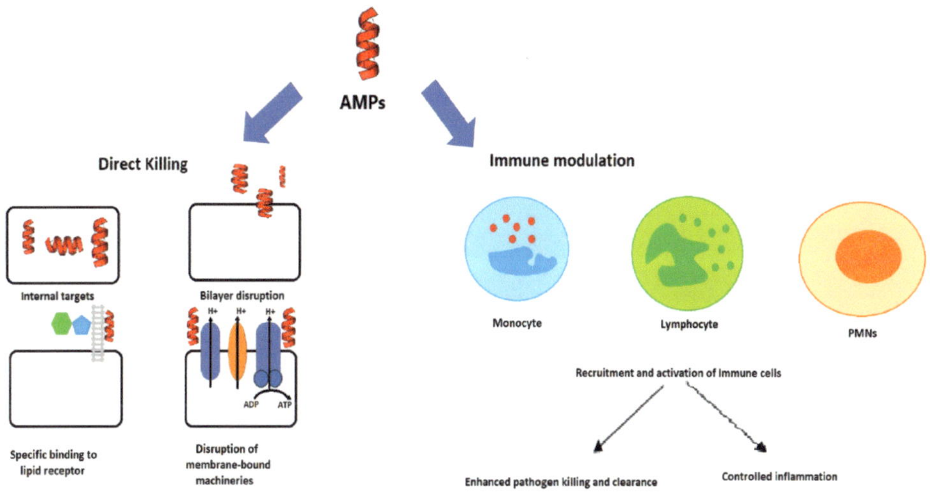

Figure 1.
Mechanism of action of antimicrobial peptides.

2.1 Direct killing: membrane targeting mechanism of action

AMPs bind through electrostatic and hydrophobic interactions to negatively charged membranes, such as bacterial outer membrane lipids with anionic head groups, like phosphatidylglycerol and cardiolipin, thereby disrupting the membranes. AMPs can interact with negatively charged membranes of microbes and display their antimicrobial activity due to the positive charge present on their α-helix surface, which play important role in killing microbes. The hydrophobic regions of AMPs only have weak interaction with the zwitterionic phospholipids in mammalian membranes. These peptides show less cytotoxicity towards eukaryotic cells since membranes of eukaryotic cells are generally neutral and composed of uncharged neutral phospholipids (like phospholipids comprising of phosphatidylcholine or phosphatidylethanolamine), sphingomyelins, and a huge concentration of cholesterol (**Figure 2**). Cholesterol decreases AMPs binding to mammalian cell membranes. The amino acid composition of AMPs decides their net charges, amphiphilic properties, and hydrophobicity, which is responsible for their crucial effects on the selective action to microbes [10]. For cellular communication, the electrostatic interaction between anionic phospholipids and cationic AMPs, as well as negatively charged bacterial membranes, is critical. In contrast, phospholipids having phosphatidylcholine head groups and sphingomyelin with a minor part of some ganglioside make up the outer surface of eukaryotic cell membranes, hence the hydrophobic contact between cationic AMPs and mammalian membranes is comparatively weak. Due to the presence of negatively charged phospholipids, there is significant contact between the hydrophobic portion of AMPs and the outer surface of bacterium membranes [13].

The membrane targeting AMPs interact through two ways: receptor-mediated mechanism or non-receptor-mediated mechanism.

2.1.1 Receptor-mediated mechanism

This is mediated by a small group of AMPs i.e., receptor-mediated peptides that consists of a receptor-binding domain and pore-forming domain [14]. They usually resist microbes in vitro at micromolar or nanomolar concentrations and works by interacting with membrane components.

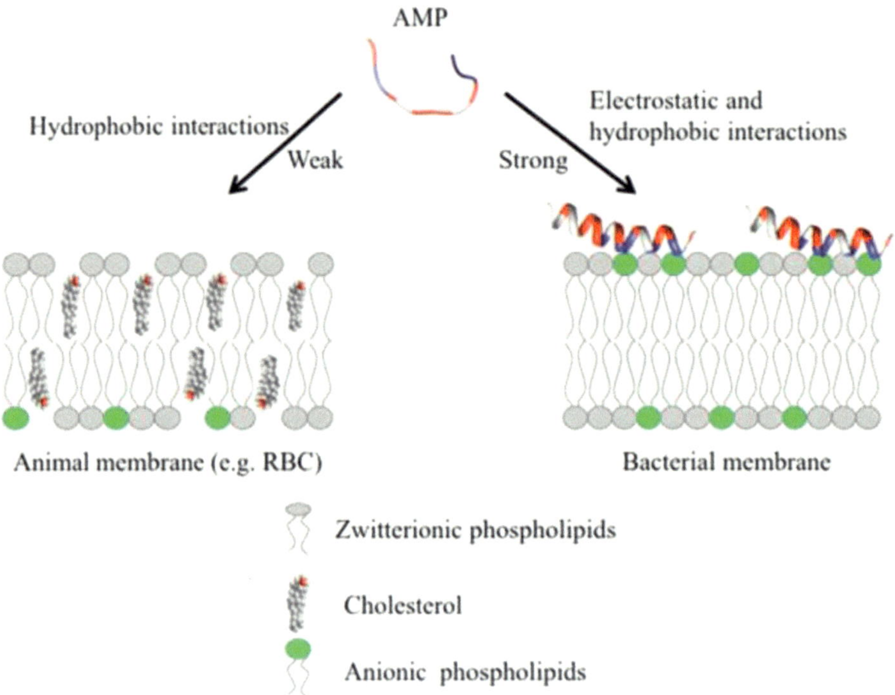

Figure 2.
AMPs' interactions with mammalian membrane or bacterial membrane [6].

This mechanism is found in the majority of AMPs generated by bacteria, viruses, and tumor cells, for example – nisin, Lacto-coccin, and mesentericin [14]. Nisin tends to be a decent example of antimicrobial activity at low concentration assisted by a definite receptor-like interaction with lipid II as a membrane-bound element concerned with peptidoglycan synthesis. Hence, nisin is reasonably more effective against peptidoglycan-rich gram-positive organisms than others [6]. It mainly comprises of two domains: the first attaches to a cell wall precursor contained in the membrane, the lipid II molecule, with high affinity and the second one is a membrane-anchored pore-forming domain. Alike Nisin, mersacidin is another AMP synthesized by Bacillus species that affiliates with the lantibiotics group. According to previous researches, mersacidin straightforwardly targets lipid II and causes interference with transglycosylation and peptidoglycan synthesis in gram-positive bacteria.

PR-39 is another example that shows a receptor-mediated mechanism to the membrane receptor SbmA. PR-39 is a cathelicidin AMP that is linear in nature and rich in proline-arginine [12]. This AMP is unable to form the pores in the bacterial membrane, although is known to possess multi-functional activities like wound healing by repressing syndecan expression, anti-inflammation via NADPH oxidase inhibition, chemoattraction for neutrophil leucocyte, and intervening protein and DNA synthesis by swift induction of proteolytic activity, prompting degeneration of some proteins involved in DNA replication [12, 15].

2.1.2 Non-receptor mediated mechanism

The non-receptor mediated action mechanism mostly includes in most vertebrate and invertebrate AMPs who exert their activity by interacting with membrane components [6]. The outer surface of the membrane of Gram-negative bacteria contains lipopolysaccharide and Gram-positive bacteria contains teichoic acid, each leads to a net negative charge on membrane surface binds with cationic AMPs through electrostatic attraction [16, 17]. The membrane permeability is the most researched mechanism to understand the MOA of AMPs. AMPs bind to microbial membranes and then destruct the membrane structures of bacteria or cancer cells, leading to the release of cell contents and resulting in cell death [12, 18–20].

In Gram-negative bacteria, the extra-cellular membrane is composed of negatively charged lipopolysaccharide (LPS). The cationic AMPs cause breakage or a cavity on the outer membranes of bacteria and finally translocate through extracellular membranes by replacing the ions such as Mg^{2+} and Ca^{2+} bound to LPS.

In contrast, Gram-positive bacteria are bounded by a single bilayer membrane which is surrounded by a cell wall containing a thick coating of peptidoglycan and lipoteichoic acid (LTA), thus creating a thick matrix that maintains the bacterial cell's stiffness. AMPs can diffuse through nano-sized pores that permeate the peptidoglycan layers [21]. LTA is a key component of cell wall of Gram-positive bacteria. It's a negatively charged molecule with a diacylglycerol moiety bound to the peptidoglycan. The presence of anionic teichoic acids in Gram-positive bacterial cell walls can potentially enhance AMP penetration by providing an extra site to interact with AMPs [14]. After penetrating through the outer membrane and single layer of peptidoglycan in Gram-negative bacteria and thick layers of peptidoglycan in Gram-positive bacteria, AMPs bind to the phospholipids which are present on the inner cellular membranes, causing the formation of a cavity on the cell membranes, thereby resulting in the destruction or permeability of cell membranes, and eventually releasing the contents of the bacteria, further bacterial cell lysis and death [22].

The mechanism of cell membrane damage comprises two steps. First, the cationic AMPs selectively bind onto the surface of the negatively charged bacterial cell membranes and then destroy bacterial membranes by either perforation or non-perforation mode. The hypothetical models which come under membrane perforation mode can be classified into four models including the barrel-stave model, the carpet model, the toroidal-pore model, and the aggregated channel model. In the non-perforation mechanism, it predicts that AMPs bind to the surface of the bacterial cell membranes to cause cell death by disrupting the normal cellular processes of the cells, such as DNA replication, RNA transcription, or protein synthesis [4].

2.2 Direct killing: non-membrane targeting mechanism of action

The non-membrane targeting MOA is broadly grouped into two major categories: AMPs that target intracellular components of bacteria and those that target the cell wall of bacteria [6].

2.2.1 Peptides who target cell wall

AMPs inhibit the synthesis of cell walls similar to traditional antibiotics via interacting with a variety of precursor molecules that are essential for cell wall formation. An example of such precursor molecule which is a main target of AMPs is lipid II [23]. For example, Peptides like defensins bind to the lipid II molecule's anionic pyrophosphate sugar moiety [24]. Due to this binding, pores formation can occur and further leads to membrane disruption [23]. Human α defensin 1 [16] and human β defensin 3 [24] are AMPs that bind to lipid II to show their bactericidal action mechanism.

2.2.2 Peptides who target Intracellular components

Many research studies indicate that AMPs can traverse the bacterial cell membranes and interact with intracellular targets such as DNA and RNA, disturbing bacterial physiological activity. This can cause interference in proteins and cell wall synthesis [17]. AMPs first interact with the cytoplasmic membrane before attacking intracellular components by inhibiting crucial cellular processes. Mechanisms that involve intracellular targets include inhibit cell-wall synthesis, inhibit the synthesis of macromolecules such as protein or nucleic acids, or inhibit enzymatic activity. Some AMPs, for example, buforin II, indolicidin translocate through and enter inside the bacterial membrane and bind to nucleic acids (DNA or RNA) and inhibit nucleic acid synthesis [6]. This mode of action is still not clear but it is assumed that the cationic amino acids of the peptides interact with the negatively charged phosphate groups of the nucleic acids electrostatically or other synthesized proteins [19]. Some AMPs now target intracellular components, as they do not produce membrane permeabilization at the minimum optimal dose yet nevertheless induce the death of bacteria [17].

2.3 Immunological regulation mechanism of action

AMPs not only directly target and destroy bacteria but may exert their antimicrobial activity by immune modulatory mechanism [20]. AMPs display their immune-modulatory effects in different ways, like reducing the endotoxin-induced inflammatory response, provoking synthesis of pro-inflammatory factors and cytokines, controlling adaptive immunity, and finally recruiting macrophages to show immune modulatory effects [25–27]. These peptides enhance the body's ability to fight microbes rather than directly killing bacteria [4].

AMPs are among the innate immunity components and they represent "the first line of defense" being one of the first molecules that fight with foreign microbes as

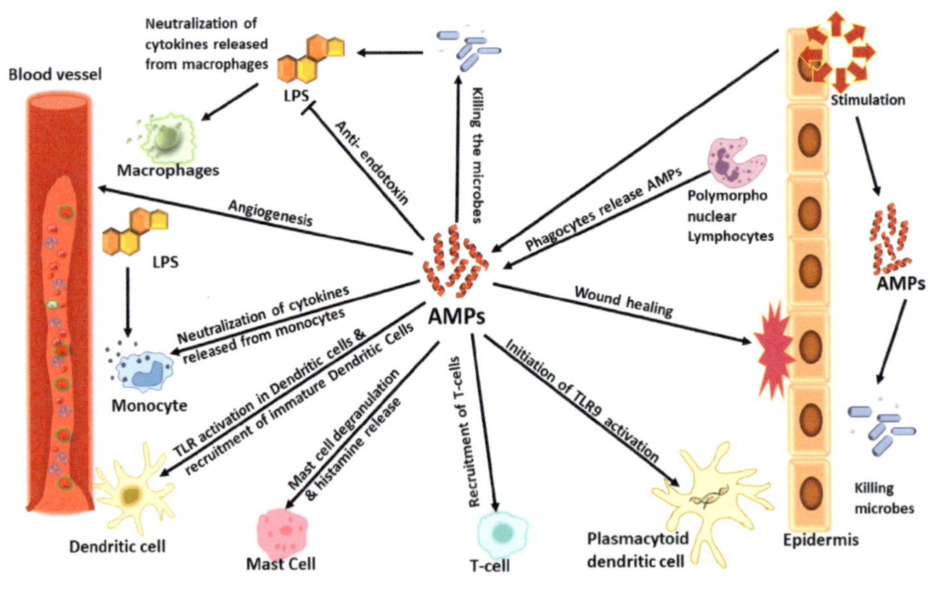

Figure 3.
AMPs affect gene expression in different cells which include macrophages, neutrophils, monocytes, and epithelial cells, and cause these cells to release chemokines and cytokines, which cause leukocytes to return to the infection site, induce cell differentiation, activate certain cells, and block or activate the Toll-like receptor signaling cascade. Infection prevention, inflammation management, healing of wounds, and provoking the defense of adaptive immunity are all aided by their actions [12].

they are produced by immunological cells like macrophages and neutrophils [28]. Some AMPs display various immune reactions like activation and differentiation of white blood cells (WBCs); reduction of expression of inflammatory chemokines; and expression management of chemokines and reactive nitrogen/oxygen species [29–33]. AMPs stimulate the immune system through various methods in mammals, viz. (i). T cell activation; (ii). Stimulation of Toll-like receptors; (iii). Elevation of phagocytosis; (iv). Dendritic cells activation; (v). chemoattraction of neutrophils (**Figure 3**) [34].

AMPs are produced by a variety of cells in the body, including epithelial cells, lymphocytes, phagocytes, neutrophils, and keratinocytes in places including the lymphatic system, genitourinary tract, gastrointestinal tract, and immune systems.

With the advancement in research studies of AMPs, it became quite evident that AMPs are produced either constitutively (frequently) or triggered by inflammation [35].

Certain immune cells including neutrophils and macrophages generate AMPs constitutively, whereas other cells like epithelial cells, produce them as a result of mucosal surface stimulation [35]. Most β-defensins are produced due to induction and AMPs that are generated frequently include α-defensins [36]. The human AMPs e.g., LL-37 and β defensins are capable of attracting immune cells like leukocytes [37], dendritic cells [38], and mast cells [25].

3. Models to describe MOA

The activity of AMPs must be considered at the cytoplasmic membrane since most of the AMPs pass through the cell membrane [26]. MOA of peptides depends upon the number of properties including the amino acids sequence, net charge, secondary structure, amphipathicity, hydrophobicity, etc. [27]. There are different mechanisms by which AMPs cause membrane disruption [39]. The capability of AMP's to bind with bacterial membrane leads to their significant development [40, 41]. There are various models hypothesized by scientists, used to describe the mechanisms of binding AMPs on a membrane including the barrel-stave, toroidal pore wormhole, carpet model as depicted in **Figure 4** [6].

The models that describe structurally less-defined mechanisms are interfacial activity, segregation of lipids into domains, non-lamellar phases formation, and the transient pore mechanism. Antimicrobial peptides' mechanism of action has been described using a variety of models. Models which are significantly applied to MOA of AMPs on the membrane are barrel stave, toroidal pore wormhole, and carpet mechanism among all the various models as depicted in **Table 1** [30, 41]. The two main pore formation models are barrel-stave and toroidal pore. The non-pore formation model is the carpet mechanism. The mechanism can be divided further into two based on cellular absorption processes: ATP dependent and ATP independent uptake process. The barrel-stave model, carpet model, or toroidal model are all ATP-independent uptake mechanisms, while macropinocytosis is an energy-dependent uptake mechanism [9]. Example of AMPs that follows energy independent cell-penetration mechanism is MMG, alamethicin and gramicidin S [9]. Example of AMP that acts through energy-dependent endocytic pathway CGA-N9 [42].

3.1 Barrel-Stave model

In the barrel-stave model, AMPs bind with the membrane outer surface via electrostatic interaction following it then undergo a conformational change attaining an amphipathic structure. Peptides with a special direction are placed between the membrane and they laterally interact with each other to form an ion channel [31].

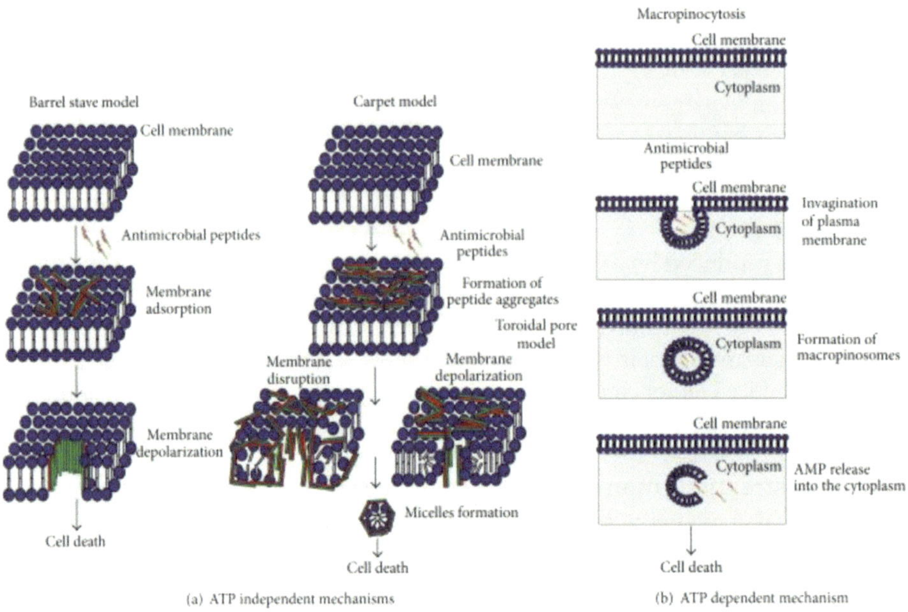

Figure 4.
Mechanism of interaction of the antimicrobial peptide with microbial membrane. (a) ATP independent cellular uptake mechanism: barrel stave model, carpet model, toroidal pore wormhole model. (b) ATP-dependent cellular uptake mechanism: macropinocytosis [9].

When peptide concentration reaches a critical threshold, the peptide monomers form an aggregate on the surface of the membrane, then they create a structure that is made up of a huge concentration of peptides inserted inside the membrane to form a ring just like a "barrel" pore. "Stave" here indicates the spokes which are contained inside the barrel [43]. The hydrophobic residues of the aggregated peptides face outward towards the hydrophobic region of the membrane, while the hydrophilic regions of the peptides face inward, forming an aqueous transmembrane pore that triggered exudation of intracellular contents and resulting death of cells [9]. Some examples of peptides that work through the barrel stave model mechanisms are alamethicin and gramicidin S [13, 44, 45]. Bioinformatic analysis of protegrin 1 conformed that the calculated energy of peptide insertion in artificial membranes was most congruent with this model (**Figure 4(a)**) [26, 33].

3.2 Toroidal pore wormhole model

The "toroidal pore wormhole" model works similarly to the "barrel stave" mechanism. The peptides are first attracted to the membrane in parallel orientation and then go through secondary structural modifications that are equivalent to those seen in the barrel stave model. The hydrophilic head of peptides faces the hydrophilic region of lipids in this arrangement, and the aqueous phase is outside of the membrane, whereas the hydrophobic portion is located in the membrane's hydrophobic core. The hydrophobic region of the peptides attach to the phospholipid head regions and displace them. This generates a rupture in the hydrophobic part of the membrane, resulting in a strain. The strain, as well as membrane thinning, creates the surface of bilayer fragile to the AMPs by destructing the composition of the membrane [33].

When the critical threshold concentration of peptides is achieved, the peptides form a self aggregate and thus create the toroidal pore complex, directing

	Models of antimicrobial action	Antimicrobial peptides
Non-permeabilizing models		
1	Transient pore model	Buforin II
2	Sinking raft model	δ-lysin
Permeabilizing models		
1	Barrel-Stave model	Alamethicin, Pardaxin 1
2	Toroidal pore model	Melittin,LL-37
3	Huge toroidal pore model	Lacticin Q
4	Disordered toroidal pore model	Melittin
5	Aggregate model	Magainins, Dermaseptin
6	Interfacial activity	Magainin 2
7	Chaotic activity	Magainin 2
8	Carpet mechanism	Aurein 1.2,Cecropin,Indolicidin
9	Membrane discrimination model	V13KL
10	Shai-Huang-Matsazuki (SHM) model	PMAP-23
11	Membrane thinning/thickening model	LL-37
12	Charged clustering of lipids	Magainin analogues
13	Sand in a gearbox model	Synthetic α-AMPs
14	Oxidized phospholipid targeting	Temporin L
15	Electroporation model	NK-lysin
16	Tilted peptide mechanism	Aurein 1.2
17	Amyloid formation model	Temporin B
18	Inhibition of synthesis of macromolecules	Indolicin, PR-39
19	Inhibition of metabolic activities	Histatins

Table 1.
Various Models for the interaction of AMPs with membrane [29, 30].

themselves in a perpendicular direction to the bilayer surface with the hydrophobic residues not accessible to the phospholipid head groups. The peptides still have an interaction with the phospholipid head regions and are not localized inside the hydrophobic region of the membrane, which distinguishes this from the barrel stave pore. Since this configuration is less stable than a barrel stave pore, thus it is more transitory. Peptide charge appears to alter the stability of pores, with a significant amount of positive side chain residues inducing repulsion and resulting in transitory pores with very short half-lives [43]. The peptides interact through electrostatic attraction with the membrane and following it undergo the same conformational alterations in the same way as the barrel stave model.

In this model, the peptides can orient themselves in a perpendicular direction too in the bilayer membrane [46], also this model does not need specific peptide–peptide interactions to occur. Instead, the peptides cause pore formation within a local curvature of the membrane which is partially formed by the phospholipid head regions. One feature which differentiates the toroidal-pore model from the barrel-stave is the complete arrangement of the lipid membrane. The hydrophobic and hydrophilic arrangement of the bilayer is kept intact in the barrel-stave mechanism, while in toroidal pores this arrangement of the lipids is disrupted, due to which a lipid head and lipid tail groups start interacting with each other. Some peptides traverse through the cytoplasmic membrane enter inside the cytoplasm and start attacking intracellular components as the pores are transient upon the destruction of the membrane [47]. Various AMPs act by toroidal pore models like magainin 2, lacticin Q, and melittin (**Figure 4(a)**) [6].

3.3 Carpet model

The carpet model, originally described by Shai [40], is the widely studied model for destabilization of the membrane by AMPs. AMPs can also perform the antimicrobial activity without pores formation in the membrane. Carpet model is one such model [17, 41, 48]. Similar to the other two models the mechanism occurs when cationic AMPs are initially attracted with strong electrostatic interaction to a negatively charged phospholipid membrane. AMPs are oriented in a parallel direction to the lipid bilayer membrane surface. Peptides accumulate themselves until they reach to critical threshold concentration, to form a "carpet" on the membrane, leading to unnecessary binding interactions on the outer surface of the membrane, thus rupture of the membrane occurs by creating an effect just like detergent, which leads to micelle formation [23]. There are a few models which can't be distinguished. The carpet model is one of them and it has been proposed as a necessary step for the toroidal pore model [30]. The membrane bilayer is broken into micelles is referred to as a detergent-like model. The carpet mechanism does not need peptide–peptide interactions of the peptide individuals bound to the membrane; nor does it need the peptide to embed itself into the hydrophobic region to create transmembrane channels [33]. Some peptides' antimicrobial activity is independent of their amino acid or sequence length; such peptides use the carpet model to demonstrate their action [41], and they perform their action when they are in large amounts because of their amphiphilicity [28]. AMPs performing their activity with the mechanism of carpet model are e.g., cecropin [49] and aurein 1.2 (**Figure 4(a)**) [50].

3.4 Other models

The models which have ATP-independent cellular uptake mechanisms involve the barrel-stave model, carpet model, or toroidal model, which we have already discussed. ATP-dependent uptake mechanism involves macropinocytosis. Macropinocytosis is the ATP-dependent uptake method of action of AMPs, where the target cell's plasma membrane folds inward along with the peptide to generate macropinosomes. Furthermore, the AMPs in the vesicles are exudated inside the cytoplasm and show the antibacterial effect (**Figure 4(b)**) [18, 45]. There are several other models by which peptides perform their antimicrobial action. In models like sinking raft and electroporation, unstable holes emerge in the membrane, altering the charge on both sides of the membrane and eventually developing holes [44].

4. Mechanism of action against other targets

Mechanism of AMPs is widely studied against other targets as well like viruses, fungi, and cancer. Gram-positive bacteria and Gram-negative bacteria are the most commonly studied targets though [2].

4.1 Anticancer antimicrobial peptides

Cancer cells are moderately anionic because of the negatively charged molecules present on their membrane-like phosphatidylserine, O-glycosylated mucins, sialylated gangliosides, and heparin sulfate [51]. In cancer cells, the asymmetry between the inner and outside membranes in terms of negatively charged phospholipids is lost, leads to an increase in negatively charged phosphatidylserine (PS) on the outer leaflet, which improves interactions with AMPs [52]. Due to these anionic molecules present on the cancer cells, electrostatic attraction occurs between cationic AMPs and anionic cancerous cells leading to membrane disruption through mechanisms like carpet or barrel-stave [53, 54].

Anticancer peptides also display anticancer activity through non-membrane targeting mechanisms (i) recruitment and activation of dendritic or macrophage cells to kill tumor cells (ii) obstructing angiogenesis to prevent tumor nutrition and metastasis (iii) inducing cancer cell necrosis or apoptosis (iv) activation of some functional proteins which interfere with tumor cell gene transcription and translation. It's worth noting that both net charge and hydrophobicity play key roles in anticancer activity optimization, and they are interdependent. For greater anticancer activity, maintaining a balance between net charge and hydrophobicity is crucial [11]. Examples of AMPs that exhibit anticancer activity are magainins and defensins [2].

4.2 Antiviral antimicrobial peptides

AMPs have been found to have inhibitory effects on a variety of DNA and RNA viruses, including HIV and influenza virus, herpes virus, and the hepatitis B virus.

AMPs have been discovered to have antiviral properties in various ways [22]. Antiviral peptides block viruses at various life cycle stages which include entry, attachment, penetration, uncoating, biosynthesis, assembly, and release. AMPs display antiviral mechanisms broadly through three ways: (i) hindering virus attachment and virus-cell membrane fusion; (ii) disrupting the virus envelope; and (iii) inhibition of virus replication by interacting with viral polymerase [12]. AMPs can potentially have an indirect antiviral effect, by altering the host immunological response. They can stimulate the synthesis of cytokines and chemokines, displaying both normal pro-inflammatory activity and triggering the infection-induced inflammatory response. AMPs may also operate as a chemoattractant, attracting immune cells to the infection site and aiding viral clearance [55]. Examples of AMPs showing antiviral activity include α-defensins interfere with the ability of the human immunodeficiency virus (HIV) to multiply within CD4 cells by directly inactivating viral particles. Retrocyclin 2 is a synthetic θ-defensin, capable of preventing influenza virus infection. Human β-defensins can prevent HIV-1 replication [26].

4.3 Antifungal antimicrobial peptides

Antifungal antimicrobial peptides attack either intracellular components or cell walls, causing fungal cell membrane integrity to be disrupted and permeability to be altered due to pore creation in the membrane structure [12]. Antifungal peptides have several recognized mechanisms of action including, (i) direct membrane disruption, (ii) inhibition of cell wall formation, primarily of components like (1,3)- β- d-glucan or chitin, and (iii) interaction with fungal mitochondria [2]. A classic example of an AFP that inhibits 1,3- β-glucan synthase is the echinocandin family. This enzyme is crucial for fungi to maintain cell wall stability. The cell wall is destabilized and the cells become vulnerable to osmotic pressure when the function of this enzyme is blocked. The β-glucan synthase enzyme is broadly found in *Aspergillus, Cryptococcus, Candida, and Pneumocystis* species. Inhibitors like nikkomycin and polyoxins are known to block chitin synthase in species like *C. albicans* [12].

5. Biophysical techniques to determine MOA

Various biophysical methods can be used to explain the MOA of AMPs. These methods depend upon bacterial components (e.g., DNA, lipid extracts, nucleotides, etc.). They provide significant insights on the MOA in-depth specifically when the MOA does not include membrane disruption.

5.1 Membrane disruption

The membrane damaging MOA has been the focal point of many researchers for many years [6]. Following are the techniques to determine membrane disrupting mechanisms.

5.1.1 Pyranine leakage assay

Pyranine (Trisodium 8-hydroxypyrene-1,3,6-trisulfonate) is a pH-sensitive hydrophilic polyanionic molecule used as a fluorescent dye to detect the quantity of internal aqueous proton in phospholipid vesicles. Pyranine and anionic phospholipid vesicles have no considerable interaction, due to the anionic nature of pyranine. These properties utilize the use of pyranine molecules to examine the transport of hydrogen ions and counterion across phospholipid vesicle membranes even in the presence of AMPs that disrupt membranes [56, 57]. The accessory information provided through this method is that leakage is affected by membrane composition or ions which are very crucial for activity, like Ca^{2+} [2].

5.1.2 Calcein leakage assay

Calcein leakage assay can be used to study the ability of AMPs to disrupt the lipid bilayers like large unilamellar vesicles (LUVs) or small unilamellar vesicles (SUVs). Calcein or carboxyfluorescein is an aqueous soluble fluorescent dye that is entrapped into LUVs and a gel filtration mechanism is used to eliminate the non-entrapped calcein after self-quenching at critical extreme concentrations [7]. If peptides cause membrane disruption or create large pores in the bilayer, this can lead to leakage of entrapped calcein out of the vesicle lumen thus relieving the self-quenching and resulting in an increase in fluorescence emission intensity [58]. This assay can also be utilized to understand the effect of AMP on bacterial cytoplasmic membrane integrity [59].

5.2 Membrane interaction

Following techniques are used to explain the mechanism of how antimicrobial peptides interact with the plasma membrane.

5.2.1 Oriented circular dichroism

It is significantly crucial to understand the interaction of AMPs with model membranes since many AMPs show their activity by traversing through the membranes. Oriented circular dichroism (OCD) is the method by which we can study the interaction. Oriented lipid bilayers are employed in OCD to gain insights into the peptide membrane alignment [7]. A clear difference between parallel vs. perpendicular localization of a peptide concerning the bilayer membrane can be observed through the signal [60]. This method is mostly studied on α-helical peptides. A change in the CD signal is observed when peptides form well-defined pores with respect to increase in peptide concentration [7].

5.2.2 Differential quenching

Differential quenching is the method that is utilized to gain insights into the localization of peptides in the lipid bilayer membrane [61]. The method takes advantage of simple diffusional quenching notions to the bilayer membrane's constrained dimensions. The membrane bilayer serves as a slab in which fluorophores and quenchers are distributed uniformly. The quenchers' distribution has been described using simulations of single-molecule Brownian dynamics, whereas the fluorophores' distribution has been determined using quenchers' pairs in phospholipids that are generally in different orientations of the acyl chain in the phospholipids [62]. Because the relative degree of quenching between quenchers and fluorophores is dependent on their propinquity, and the information on the peptides' current location in the membrane will be provided by fluorescence intensity [61]. A water-soluble quencher, like acrylamide, can also be employed to detect whether the fluorophore is not affected by the aqueous conditions, which is a useful addition to this assay [63].

5.2.3 Other methods

Several other methods like differential scanning calorimetry (DSC) and ^{2}H or ^{31}P solid-state NMR can be used to examine how antimicrobial peptides affect lipid arrangement. The DSC thermogram does not show any alterations in AMPs that traverse through the membrane. Alteration in phosphorus nuclei orientation in the membrane depends upon alteration in ^{31}P chemical shift, and this also gives accessory information on AMP mode of action. ^{2}H NMR analyses the effect of the AMP on the order of the acyl chain. Currently, DSC is utilized to examine the binding of the AMP MSI-78 with bacteria. Similarly, ^{31}P NMR is used to detect the whole bacterial cells [7].

5.3 Nucleic acid interaction

Gel electrophoresis can be used to examine the interaction of AMPs with nucleic acids. The mobility of the nucleic acid bands (Deoxyribonucleic acid (DNA) or Ribonucleic acid (RNA)) is typically measured with respect to AMP concentration. When AMP binds to DNA, the band migration rate is reduced or completely inhibited [64]. Ethidium bromide is used to stain the bands, it is an intercalating agent which can insert itself between nitrogenous base pairs in the DNA, thus used as nucleic acid fluorescent tag and detected by Ultraviolet light. For instance, the nucleic acid binding activity of AMP such as buforin II kills *E. coli* cells quickly without lysis, detected by the agarose gel electrophoresis technique [7].

5.4 Nucleotide interaction

AMPs show interaction with nucleotides like Adenosine triphosphate (ATP) [65]. In biofilms, one such crucial mechanism for AMPs is to interact with the alarmone nucleotides (p) ppGpp which can be detected by a co-precipitation assay. This interaction results in ppGpp degradation in bacteria, blocking the stress reaction, which further results in the prevention of biofilms or removal of already formed biofilms [7].

5.5 Other methods

Several other methods include determining different types of interactions, for instance, the capacity of AMPs to interact with protein molecules to prevent the formation of biofilm [66]. The co-precipitation method can be used, to detect the capability of AMPs to interact with proteins. For example, the ribosomal protein binding activity of Bac71–35 was examined by measuring the activity of co-sedimentation of ribosomes that have been purified with Bac71–35. After incubating *E. coli* 70S ribosomes with various doses of the peptide, the peptide bound to the ribosome was isolated using ultracentrifugation. Immunoblotting was used to validate the existence of Ba71–35 and ribosomal protein interaction in the ribosomal pellets [56].

Alternatively, the presence of peptide can be detected by labeling it with rhodamine whether the peptide is on the membrane surface of bacteria or inside the bacteria or on a solid attachment [66] or fluorescent dyes [57]. It is crucial to confirm that the label should not cause any interference with the activity and composition of peptides. Finally, several other kinds of interactions (for instance, lipid II or LPS) can be detected by the use of techniques such as Nuclear Magnetic Resonance (NMR) or surface plasmon resonance (SPR) [7].

6. Conclusion

Antimicrobial peptides are an essential component of innate immunity. They have the potential to be a viable alternative to antibiotics. It is critical to comprehend the MOA used by AMPs to kill bacteria to increase their development as therapeutics. The selectivity and activity of these peptides are influenced by a variety of parameters. Properties such as net charge, hydrophobicity, secondary structure, and amphipathicity are all important for function and are so interconnected that changing one attribute generally causes alterations in others.

The AMPs aggregate at the membrane surface following the hydrophobic and electrostatic attraction, forming self-aggregate on the bacterial membrane after they reach a particular concentration. The MOA of peptides can be broadly divided into two classes including direct killing and immunological regulation, wherein direct killing is further categorized into membrane targeting and non-membrane targeting. Different models have been proposed to explain the mechanism of interaction of peptides with membranes. Some biophysical techniques are used to determine their action mechanism whether these peptides disrupt microbial membrane or they target intracellular activities. Therefore, it is very crucial to know about the diverse biological features of AMPs for their clinical development.

DOI: http://dx.doi.org/10.5772/intechopen.99190

Author details

Tanu Singh, Princy Choudhary and Sangeeta Singh*
Applied Science Department, Indian Institute of Information Technology, Allahabad, India

*Address all correspondence to: sangeeta@iiita.ac.in

References

[1] Kościuczuk EM, Lisowski P, Jarczak J, Strzałkowska N, Jóźwik A, Horbańczuk J, et al. Cathelicidins: family of antimicrobial peptides. A review. Mol Biol Rep. 2012 Dec; 39 (12): 10957-10970.

[2] Zhang LJ, Gallo RL. Antimicrobial peptides. Curr Biol [Internet]. 2016; 26(1): R14-9. Available from: doi:10. 1016/j.cub.2015.11.017

[3] Benfield AH, Henriques ST. Mode-of-Action of Antimicrobial Peptides: Membrane Disruption vs. Intracellular Mechanisms. Front Med Technol. 2020 Dec 11; 2.

[4] Lei J, Sun LC, Huang S, Zhu C, Li P, He J, et al. The antimicrobial peptides and their potential clinical applications. Am J Transl Res. 2019; 11(7): 3919-3931.

[5] Le C-F, Fang C-M, Sekaran SD. Intracellular Targeting Mechanisms by Antimicrobial Peptides. Antimicrob Agents Chemother. 2017 Apr;61(4).

[6] Kumar P, Kizhakkedathu JN, Straus SK. Antimicrobial peptides: Diversity, mechanism of action and strategies to improve the activity and biocompatibility in vivo. Biomolecules. 2018;8(1).

[7] Raheem N, Straus SK. Mechanisms of Action for Antimicrobial Peptides With Antibacterial and Antibiofilm Functions. Front Microbiol. 2019;10(December):1-14.

[8] Li J, Koh JJ, Liu S, Lakshminarayanan R, Verma CS, Beuerman RW. Membrane active antimicrobial peptides: Translating mechanistic insights to design. Front Neurosci. 2017;11(FEB):1-18.

[9] Pushpanathan M, Gunasekaran P, Rajendhran J. Antimicrobial peptides: Versatile biological properties. Int J Pept. 2013;2013(Table 1).

[10] Jäkel CE, Meschenmoser K, Kim Y, Weiher H, Schmidt-Wolf IGH. Efficacy of a proapoptotic peptide towards cancer cells. In Vivo (Brooklyn). 2012;26(3):419-426.

[11] Huan Y, Kong Q, Mou H, Yi H. Antimicrobial Peptides: Classification, Design, Application and Research Progress in Multiple Fields. Front Microbiol. 2020;11(October):1-21.

[12] Moravej H, Moravej Z, Yazdanparast M, Heiat M, Mirhosseini A, Moosazadeh Moghaddam M, et al. Antimicrobial Peptides: Features, Action, and Their Resistance Mechanisms in Bacteria. Microb Drug Resist. 2018;24(6):747-767.

[13] Seyfi R, Kahaki FA, Ebrahimi T, Montazersaheb S, Eyvazi S, Babaeipour V, et al. Antimicrobial Peptides (AMPs): Roles, Functions and Mechanism of Action. Int J Pept Res Ther [Internet]. 2020;26(3):1451-63. Available from: https://doi.org/10.1007/s10989-019-09946-9

[14] Zhang LJ, Gallo RL. Antimicrobial peptides. Vol. 26, Current Biology. 2016. 14-19 p.

[15] Huang Y, Huang J, Chen Y. Alpha-helical cationic antimicrobial peptides: relationships of structure and function. Protein Cell. 2010 Feb;1(2):143-152.

[16] de Leeuw E, Li C, Zeng P, Li C, Diepeveen-de Buin M, Lu W-Y, et al. Functional interaction of human neutrophil peptide-1 with the cell wall precursor lipid II. FEBS Lett. 2010 Apr;584(8):1543-1548.

[17] Brogden KA. Antimicrobial peptides: Pore formers or metabolic

inhibitors in bacteria? Nat Rev Microbiol. 2005;3(3):238-250.

[18] Som A, Vemparala S, Ivanov I, Tew G. Synthetic mimics of antimicrobial peptides. Biopolymers. 2008 Jan 1;90:83-93.

[19] GuangShun W. Antimicrobial peptides: discovery, design and novel therapeutic strategies. Wallingford: CABI; 2017. xvii + 268 pp.

[20] Zasloff M. Antimicrobial Peptides of Multicellular Organisms: My Perspective. Adv Exp Med Biol. 2019;1117:3-6.

[21] Meroueh SO, Bencze KZ, Hesek D, Lee M, Fisher JF, Stemmler TL, et al. Three-dimensional structure of the bacterial cell wall peptidoglycan. Proc Natl Acad Sci U S A. 2006;103(12): 4404-4409.

[22] Lei J, Sun L, Huang S, Zhu C, Li P, He J, et al. The antimicrobial peptides and their potential clinical applications. Am J Transl Res. 2019;11(7):3919-3931.

[23] Lohner K. Membrane-active Antimicrobial Peptides as Template Structures for Novel Antibiotic Agents. Curr Top Med Chem. 2017;17(5): 508-519.

[24] Münch D, Sahl H-G. Structural variations of the cell wall precursor lipid II in Gram-positive bacteria - Impact on binding and efficacy of antimicrobial peptides. Biochim Biophys Acta. 2015 Nov;1848(11 Pt B):3062-71.

[25] Niyonsaba F, Iwabuchi K, Someya A, Hirata M, Matsuda H, Ogawa H, et al. A cathelicidin family of human antibacterial peptide LL-37 induces mast cell chemotaxis. Immunology. 2002 May;106(1):20-26.

[26] Conde R, Arguello M, Izquierdo J, Noguez R, Moreno M, Lanz H. Natural Antimicrobial Peptides from Eukaryotic Organisms. Antimicrob Agents. 2012;

[27] Mojsoska B, Zuckermann R, Jenssen H. Structure-Activity Relationship Study of Novel Peptoids That Mimic the Structure of Antimicrobial Peptides. Antimicrob Agents Chemother. 2015 May 4;59.

[28] Jenssen H, Hamill P, Hancock REW. Peptide antimicrobial agents. Clin Microbiol Rev. 2006 Jul;19(3):491-511.

[29] Juretić D, Vukičević D, Tossi A. Tools for Designing Amphipathic Helical Antimicrobial Peptides. Methods Mol Biol. 2017;1548:23-34.

[30] Lee T-H, Hall KN, Aguilar M-I. Antimicrobial Peptide Structure and Mechanism of Action: A Focus on the Role of Membrane Structure. Curr Top Med Chem. 2016;16(1):25-39.

[31] Harder J, Schröder J-M. Antimicrobial peptides: role in human health and disease. Springer; 2015.

[32] He K, Ludtke SJ, Worcester DL, Huang HW. Neutron scattering in the plane of membranes: structure of alamethicin pores. Biophys J [Internet]. 1996;70(6):2659-2666. Available from: http://europepmc.org/abstract/MED/8744303

[33] Yeaman MR, Yount NY. Mechanisms of antimicrobial peptide action and resistance. Pharmacol Rev. 2003 Mar;55(1):27-55.

[34] Matejuk A, Leng Q, Begum MD, Woodle MC, Scaria P, Chou S-T, et al. Peptide-based Antifungal Therapies against Emerging Infections. Drugs Future [Internet]. 2010 Mar;35(3):197. Available from: https://pubmed.ncbi.nlm.nih.gov/20495663

[35] Stevenson C, Marshall L, Morgan D. Progress in Inflammation Research

[Internet]. Researchgate.Net. 2006. 216 p. Available from: http://www.researchgate.net/publication/227227937_The_paleolithic_disease-scape_the_hygiene_hypothesis_and_the_second_epidemiological_transition/file/e0b495179ba29d129e.pdf

[36] Ganz T. Defensins: antimicrobial peptides of innate immunity. Nat Rev Immunol. 2003 Sep;3(9):710-720.

[37] García JR, Jaumann F, Schulz S, Krause A, Rodríguez-Jiménez J, Forssmann U, et al. Identification of a novel, multifunctional beta-defensin (human beta-defensin 3) with specific antimicrobial activity. Its interaction with plasma membranes of Xenopus oocytes and the induction of macrophage chemoattraction. Cell Tissue Res. 2001 Nov;306(2):257-264.

[38] Liu Y-J. Dendritic Cell Subsets and Lineages, and Their Functions in Innate and Adaptive Immunity. Cell [Internet]. 2001 Aug 10;106(3):259-62. Available from: https://doi.org/10.1016/S0092-8674(01)00456-1

[39] Mahlapuu M, Håkansson J, Ringstad L, Björn C. Antimicrobial Peptides: An Emerging Category of Therapeutic Agents [Internet]. Vol. 6, Frontiers in Cellular and Infection Microbiology. 2016. p. 194. Available from: https://www.frontiersin.org/article/10.3389/fcimb.2016.00194

[40] Gazit E, Miller IR, Biggin PC, Sansom MS, Shai Y. Structure and orientation of the mammalian antibacterial peptide cecropin P1 within phospholipid membranes. J Mol Biol. 1996 May;258(5):860-870.

[41] Shai Y. Mode of action of membrane active antimicrobial peptides. Biopolymers. 2002;66(4):236-248.

[42] Li R, Chen C, Zhu S, Wang X, Yang Y, Shi W, et al. CGA-N9, an antimicrobial peptide derived from chromogranin A: direct cell penetration of and endocytosis by Candida tropicalis. Biochem J [Internet]. 2019 Feb 5;476(3):483-497. Available from: https://pubmed.ncbi.nlm.nih.gov/30610128

[43] Lee T-H, N. Hall K, Aguilar M-I. Antimicrobial Peptide Structure and Mechanism of Action: A Focus on the Role of Membrane Structure. Curr Top Med Chem. 2015;16(1):25-39.

[44] Miao J, Chen F, Duan S, Gao X, Liu G, Chen Y, et al. iTRAQ-Based Quantitative Proteomic Analysis of the Antimicrobial Mechanism of Peptide F1 against *Escherichia coli*. J Agric Food Chem [Internet]. 2015 Aug 19;63(32):7190-7. Available from: https://doi.org/10.1021/acs.jafc.5b00678

[45] Kornspan JD, Rottem S. The Phospholipid Profile of Mycoplasmas. Smith TK, editor. J Lipids [Internet]. 2012;2012:640762. Available from: https://doi.org/10.1155/2012/640762

[46] Wimley WC. Describing the mechanism of antimicrobial peptide action with the interfacial activity model. ACS Chem Biol. 2010 Oct;5(10):905-917.

[47] Uematsu N, Matsuzaki K. Polar Angle as a Determinant of Amphipathic <em>α</em>-Helix-Lipid Interactions: A Model Peptide Study. Biophys J [Internet]. 2000 Oct 1;79(4):2075-83. Available from: https://doi.org/10.1016/S0006-3495(00)76455-1

[48] Clement NR, Gould JM. Pyranine (8-hydroxy-1,3,6-pyrenetrisulfonate) as a probe of internal aqueous hydrogen ion concentration in phospholipid vesicles. Biochemistry. 1981 Mar;20(6):1534-1538.

[49] Sitaram N, Nagaraj R. Interaction of antimicrobial peptides with biological and model membranes: structural and

charge requirements for activity. Biochim Biophys Acta - Biomembr [Internet]. 1999;1462(1):29-54. Available from: https://www.sciencedirect.com/science/article/pii/S0005273699001996

[50] Fernandez DI, Le Brun AP, Whitwell TC, Sani M-A, James M, Separovic F. The antimicrobial peptide aurein 1.2 disrupts model membranes via the carpet mechanism. Phys Chem Chem Phys. 2012 Dec;14(45): 15739-15751.

[51] Schweizer F. Cationic amphiphilic peptides with cancer-selective toxicity. Eur J Pharmacol. 2009 Dec;625(1-3):190-194.

[52] Bevers EM, Comfurius P, Zwaal RF. Regulatory mechanisms in maintenance and modulation of transmembrane lipid asymmetry: pathophysiological implications. Lupus. 1996 Oct;5(5): 480-487.

[53] Oren Z, Shai Y. Mode of action of linear amphipathic alpha-helical antimicrobial peptides. Biopolymers. 1998;47(6):451-463.

[54] van Zoggel H, Carpentier G, Dos Santos C, Hamma-Kourbali Y, Courty J, Amiche M, et al. Antitumor and Angiostatic Activities of the Antimicrobial Peptide Dermaseptin B2. PLoS One [Internet]. 2012 Sep 20;7(9):e44351. Available from: https://doi.org/10.1371/journal.pone.0044351

[55] Chessa C, Bodet C, Jousselin C, Wehbe M, Lévêque N, Garcia M. Antiviral and Immunomodulatory Properties of Antimicrobial Peptides Produced by Human Keratinocytes [Internet]. Vol. 11, Frontiers in Microbiology. 2020. p. 1155. Available from: https://www.frontiersin.org/article/10.3389/fmicb.2020.01155

[56] Mardirossian M, Grzela R, Giglione C, Meinnel T, Gennaro R, Mergaert P, et al. The host antimicrobial peptide Bac71-35 binds to bacterial ribosomal proteins and inhibits protein synthesis. Chem Biol. 2014;21(12):1639-1647.

[57] Okuda K, Zendo T, Sugimoto S, Iwase T, Tajima A, Yamada S, et al. Effects of bacteriocins on methicillin-resistant Staphylococcus aureus biofilm. Antimicrob Agents Chemother. 2013;57(11):5572-5579.

[58] Chrom CL, Renn LM, Caputo GA. Characterization and antimicrobial activity of amphiphilic peptide ap3 and derivative sequences. Antibiotics. 2019;8(1):1-17.

[59] Miyoshi N, Isogai E, Hiramatsu K, Sasaki T. Activity of tick antimicrobial peptide from Ixodes persulcatus (persulcatusin) against cell membranes of drug-resistant Staphylococcus aureus. J Antibiot (Tokyo). 2017;70(2):142-146.

[60] Bürck J, Wadhwani P, Fanghänel S, Ulrich AS. Oriented circular dichroism: a method to characterize membrane-active peptides in oriented lipid bilayers. Acc Chem Res. 2016;49(2):184-192.

[61] Fernandes MX, de la Torre JG, Castanho M. Joint determination by Brownian dynamics and fluorescence quenching of the in-depth location profile of biomolecules in membranes. Anal Biochem. 2002;307(1):1-12.

[62] Matos PM, Franquelim HG, Castanho MARB, Santos NC. Quantitative assessment of peptide–lipid interactions.: Ubiquitous fluorescence methodologies. Biochim Biophys Acta (BBA)-Biomembranes. 2010;1798(11):1999-2012.

[63] Torcato IM, Castanho MARB, Henriques ST. The Application of Biophysical Techniques to Study Antimicrobial Peptides. Spectrosc An Int J [Internet]. 2012;27:460702.

Available from: https://doi.org/10.1155/2012/460702

[64] Nam B-H, Moon J-Y, Park E-H, Kim Y-O, Kim D-G, Kong HJ, et al. Antimicrobial activity of peptides derived from olive flounder lipopolysaccharide binding protein/bactericidal permeability-increasing protein (LBP/BPI). Mar Drugs. 2014;12(10):5240-5257.

[65] Hilpert K, McLeod B, Yu J, Elliott MR, Rautenbach M, Ruden S, et al. Short cationic antimicrobial peptides interact with ATP. Antimicrob Agents Chemother. 2010;54(10):4480-4483.

[66] Segev-Zarko L, Saar-Dover R, Brumfeld V, Mangoni ML, Shai Y. Mechanisms of biofilm inhibition and degradation by antimicrobial peptides. Biochem J. 2015;468(2):259-270.

Chapter 4

Antimicrobial Peptides Derived from Ascidians and Associated Cyanobacteria

Rajaian Pushpabai Rajesh and Grace Vanathi M

Abstract

Ascidians belonging to Phylum Chordata are the most largest and diverse of the Sub-phylum Tunicata (Urochordata). Marine ascidians are one of the richest sources of bioactive peptides. These bioactive peptides from marine ascidians are confined to various types of structures such as cyclic peptides, acyclic peptides (depsipeptides), linear helical peptides with abundance of one amino acid (proline, trytophane, histidine), peptides forming hairpin like beta sheets or α-helical/β-sheet mixed structures stabilized by intra molecular disulfide bonding. Cyanobactins are fabricated through the proteolytic cleavage and cyclization of precursor peptides coupled with further posttranslational modifications such as hydroxylation, glycosylation, heterocyclization, oxidation, or prenylation of amino acids. Ascidians are known to be a rich source of bioactive alkaloids. β-carbolines form a large group of tryptophan derived antibiotics. Pyridoacridines from ascidians are tetra- or penta- cyclic aromatic alkaloids with broad range of bioactivities. Didemnidines derived from ascidian symbiotic microbes are inhibitors of phospholipase A2 and induce cell apoptosis. Meridianins are indulged in inhibiting various protein kinases such as, cyclindependent kinases, glycogen synthase kinase-3, cyclic nucleotide dependent kinases, casein kinase, and also implicate their activity of interfering with topoisomerase, altering the mitochondrial membrane potential and binding to the DNA minor groove to inhibit transcriptional activation. Most of these bioactive compounds from ascidians are already in different phases of the clinical and pre-clinical trials. They can be used for their nutraceutical values because of their antineoplastic, antihypertensive, antioxidant, antimicrobial, cytotoxic, antibacterial, antifungal, insecticidal, anti-HIV and anti-parasitic, anti-malarial, anti-trypanosomal, anti-cancer etc. This chapter mostly deals with antibacterial compounds from ascidian and their associate symbiotic cyanobacteria.

Keywords: Ascidians, Chordata, depsipeptides, β-carbolines, pyridoacridines

1. Introduction

Ascidians commonly known as tunicates or sea squirts are soft bodied and sessile animals belonging to subphylum urochordates. Sac like sea squirt ascidians produce many toxic nitrogen bearing secondary metabolites that are implicated in their chemical defense [1]. Ascidians belonging to family *Didemnidae, Prochloron* species symbiotic bacteria produce a variety of toxic and cyclic peptides known as cyanobactins [2]. Ascidians of this family have yielded structurally unique and pharmacological compounds such as didemnenones, enterocins, paterallazoles, varacins and virenamides [3]. Didemnin, isolated at first from the Caribbean tunicate *Trididemnin solidum*. Didemnin B capable of antiproliferative activity against human cancer cell lines. Didemnin B inhibits the synthesis of RNA, DNA and proteins [4]. It is found that Didemnin B being the first natural marine derived peptide to be evaluated in clinical trials, because of its dose-dependent and tolerable toxicity profiles. Toxicity profile of Didemnin B with dose dependent nausea and vomiting are the most commonly mentioned side effects [4]. However at the higher doses, Didemnin B causes severe cardiotoxicity.

Aplidine is a cyclodepsipeptide has sufficient activity against a variety of human cancer cell lines such as breast, melanoma and lung cancers [5]. Aplidine has several functional activities such as Inhibition of protein synthesis, cell cycle arrest, induction of apoptosis on cancer cells and inhibition of vascular endothelial growth factor gene. Its actions on causing cytotoxicity, involves the inhibition of ornithine decarboxylase, an enzyme that is responsible for the tumor formation and tumor growth [6]. Its approval on Phase-I clinical trial, induces on its minor toxicity tolerance limit with most of its side effects corresponding to asthenia, nausea, vomiting and transient transaminitis etc. [7].

Mollamides being a cyclodepsipeptide has suitable cytotoxic activity against a wide range of cancer cell lines such as human lung carcinoma and human colon carcinoma [8].

Trunkamide A, a cyclodepsipeptide with a thiazoline ring similar to mollamide, show antitumor activity under preclinical trials [9]. This peptide contains the thiazoline-based proline on doubly prenylated cyclopeptides. Heterocyclic amino acids such as the tryptophan and histidine also forms the part of proline rich cyclic peptides structures such as wainunuamide, phakellistatin 15,17 and stylissatin B.

However, recently pharmaceutical industries are gaining more insights on antimicrobial peptides due to their increased efficacy, high specificity, low toxicity, decreased drug interaction and direct attacking properties.

2. Alkaloids

Alkaloids are providing the majority of ascidian originating bioactive compounds. They represent a highly diverse group of compounds containing cyclic structures having a basic nitrogen atom incorporated within it. Ascidians on the other hand are produces of large quantity of alkaloids and modified peptides which exhibit a wide range of biological properties such as, Cytotoxicity, antibiotic, immunosuppressive activities, inhibition of topoisomerases (TOPO), cyclin kinase, display antimicrobial and anticancer activities by inhibiting kinase activity, including protein kinase B (PKB), Cyclin dependent kinases (CDKs), altering mitochondrial membrane potential and binding to the DNA minor groove to inhibit transcriptional activation [10].

Investigations on the biosynthesis of secondary metabolites provide evidence on the *de-novo* biosynthesis by ascidians [11]. Ascidians are a source of nitrogen bearing secondary metabolites with a varied range of biological activities. Many biological active compounds have been isolated from ascidians, it is still unclear whether this animal or associated microbial symbionts such as bacterial or fungi are true sources for the synthesis of biosynthetic metabolites.

A specific biosynthetic source of the alkaloids such as, granulatimide and isogranulatimides by specifically localizing these compounds lying inside ascidians.

Granulatimide stored in *Didemnum granulatum* tunic bladder cells were analyzed by confocal fluorescence microscopy at the granulatimide emission range, indicated the presence of fluorescent cells as highly vacuolated cells found to be dispersed in ascidian tunic [12]. Thus, this is the most exposed ascidian tissue, it pertains to show that this alkaloids may have a protective role.

2.1 Didemnidines

Didemnidines A and B are two indole spermidine alkaloids isolated from ascidian Didemnum species. Didemnidines A and B are both active as inhibitors of phospholipase A2, farnesyltransferase enzyme without cytotoxicity. It has moderate cytotoxicity towards malarial parasite, L6 cells and inhibition parasite proliferation. Antiparasitic activity of didemnidine B provides the opportunity to explore the didemnidines as antimalarial and antitrypanosomal agents [13].

2.2 Meridianins

Meridianins are brominated 3-(2-aminopyrimidine)-indoles isolated from the ascidian *Aplidium meridianum* [14]. As these meridianins are structurally similar to variolins, meridianins are identified as a promising kinase inhibitory scaffolds, which inhibits various protein kinases such as, Cyclin dependent kinases, glycogen synthase kinase 3, cyclin nucleotide dependent kinases and casein kinase [15].

2.3 Herdmanines

Herdmanines represent a series of nucleoside derivatives isolated from the ascidian *Herdmania monus*. Herdmanines A to D inhibit the production and the expression of messanger RNA, Pro-inflammatory cytokines, while herdmanines C and D are found to have moderate suppressive effects on the pro-inflammatory cytokines and lipopolysaccharides (LPS) induced nitricoxide [16].

2.4 Ecteinascidins

This peptide belonging to tetrahydroisoquinoline alkaloid family exhibits potent antitumor activity. It binds with the major groove of DNA and leads to the sequence specific alterations in transcription, triggers DNA cleavage, causing double stranded break, interruption of the cell cycle, apoptosis of cancer cell and down regulation of some transcriptional [17] factors.

2.5 Eusynstyelamides

Eusynstyelaides, alkaloids isolated from ascidian *Eusynstye latatericus*. It has specific cytotoxic activity against neuronal nitric oxide synthase (nNOS), anticancer and antibacterial activities. Eusynstyelaides B, a secondary metabolite from a bryozoan species, suggested that these components could be synthesized by symbiotic microbes. Eusynstyelaides B exhibits anti-proliferative activity and causes a strong cell cycle block and also induces cell apoptosis [18]. Eusynstyelamides A–C show specific cytotoxicity against neuronal nitric oxide synthase (nNOS) and show anticancer and antibacterial activity [19]. Eusynstyelamides A and B display, inhibitory activities against *Staphylococcus aureus*, plant regulatory enzymes pyruvate phosphate dikinase (PPDK) [20].

2.6 Sesbanimide

Sesbanimide A, peptide isolated from Agrobacterium. Sesbanimide C showed activity against the growth of mouse leukemia cells and inhibited the proliferation of mouth epidermal carcinoma (kb) cell [21]. It was evaluated against various human cancer cell lines.

2.7 Mollamide

A cyclodepsipeptide isolated from the ascidian *Didemnum molle*, shows specific cytotoxic activity towards a range of cell lines with IC 50 values of 1ug/ml towards P388murine leukemia cell lines and 2.5ug/ml resistance towards A549 human lung carcinoma and HT29 human colon carcinoma [22]. Neuromuscular toxicity with the elevation of creatine phosphatase levels has been dose limited, but seemed to be readily irreversible with oral carnitine. Aplidine has shown antitumor activity in phase-I clinical trials and in phase-II clinical trials in solid tumors.

3. Antimicrobial peptides from ascidians

Peptides are one of the major structural classes isolated from ascidians, including linear peptides, depsipeptides, and cyclic peptides, with residue numbers spanning from two to forty eight. Most of the active peptides from ascidians have complex cyclic of linear structures rarely found in terrestrial animals. These peptides are found to affect cell behavior with different mechanisms such as apoptosis, affecting the tubulin- microtubule environment and [23] inhibiting angiogenesis.

3.1 Vitilevuamide

A bicyclic peptide isolated from ascidian *Didemnum cuculiferum* and *Polysyncranton lithostrotum*. It was found that Vitilevuamide show activity against mouse lymphocytic leukemia. Its mechanism of cytotoxicity is due to its inhibition of tubulin polymerization without competitive inhibition of the vinblastine binding site, affects GTP binding to tubulin and also cell cycle arrest in the G2/M phase (**Figure 1**).

3.2 Diazonamides

A group of macrocytic peptides isolated from the ascidians *Diazona angulate*. Amoung various diazolzmides, Diazolamide A was evaluated for its antitumor activities [24]. It is a tubulin binding agent which blocks the cell cycle in G2/M period. Diazonamides A is a potentially chemotherapeutic agent without significant toxicity on animal models [25].

3.3 Chondromodulin-1 (ChM-1)

Chondromodulin, a 25kD a glycoprotein isolated from fetal bovine cartilage. Recently, Chondromodulin isolated from the invertebrate ascidian *Ciona savignyl*. It promotes the proliferation of mouse osteoblastic cell and also protects the H2O2 oxidation injury. Chondromodulin also modifies the cell behavior through regulating the cell cycle and cell adhesion [26]. It was found that Chondromodulin acts as a potential antioxidant and antitumor agent [27].

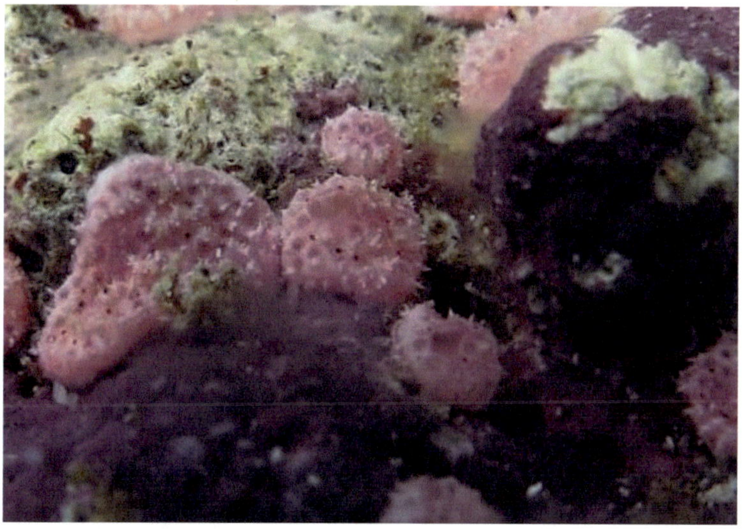

Figure 1.
Image showing Didemnum cuculiferum.

4. Polypeptide from ascidian associated microbes

4.1 Patellamides

Patellamides are cyclic peptides isolated from the cyanobacterium *Lissoclinum patella*. Patellamides A, C, D exhibits cytotoxic effects. Patellamides A and C inhibit the growth of murine leukemia cells, while patellamide D acts as a resistance modifying agent in the multidrug resistant human leukemia cell lines [28].

4.2 Polyketides

Polyketides are the other important compounds in the screening of secondary metabolites. Polyketides are complex molecules built from simple carboxylic acids and synthesized by polyketide synthetase [29]. Polyketides has been discovered as important lead compounds with various activities, such as blocking protein tyrosine phosphatase and inhibiting ATP synthetase complex [30]. Highly cytotoxic patellazole A, thought to have a defensive role, is a polyketide peptide hybrid made by the alpha-proteobacterium Ca. *Endolissoclinum faulkneri*. This bacteria was found only in a subgroup of *Lissoclinum patella*, and its genome is extensively reduced, that the bacteria is only found in a subgroup of *Lissoclinum patella*, and its genome is reduced, such that it cannot live independently in a host. These peptides are known to maintain all the synthesized genes, providing evidence for an essential defensive role of these metabolites in this symbiotic relationship [31].

4.3 Mandelalides

Mandelalides A-D are macrocyclic polyketides isolated from a new species *Lissoclinum mandelai* in south Africa. Mandelalides are glycosylated polyketides isolated from ascidian *Lissoclinum* (**Figure 2**). Mandelalides A and B show potent cytotoxicity towards, NCI-H460 cells and mouse Neuro-2a neuroblastoma cells. Mandelalides B display potent antifungicidal activity against *Candida albicans* [32]. Isomandelalide A exhibited unexpectedly high level of activity being more potent than mandelalide B. Glycosylated mandelalides A and B are cytotoxic to

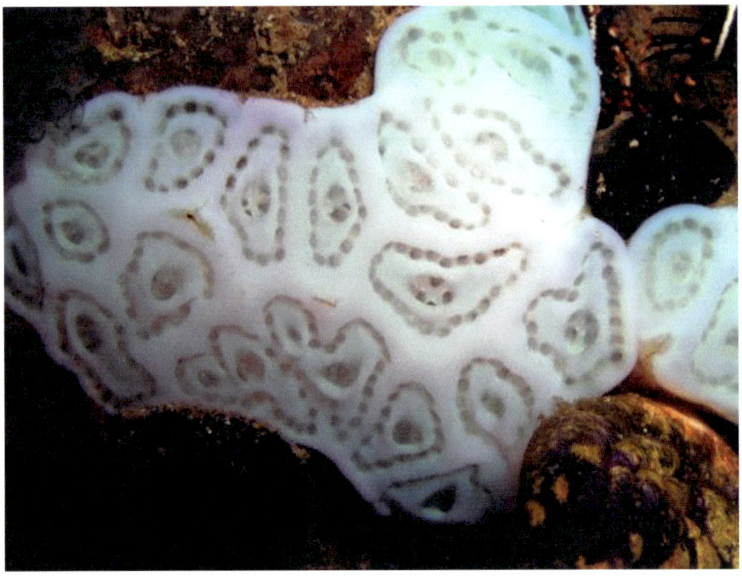

Figure 2.
Image showing cyanobacterium Lissoclinum patella.

neuroblastoma cells at low nanomolecular concentrations. New mandelalides G-L isolated allowing the activity of structure activity relationship, comparing the activities of monoscharrides and macrocyclic acylation on biological activity. The structures of Mandelalidea A and B are shown in the figure. Cytotoxic activity of mandelalide A was dependent on cell density with actively proliferating tumor cells at low density being actively resistant to the compound. Mandelalides A and B inhibited mitochondrial function and induce caspase dependent apoptotic cell death, due to the inhibition of the mammalian ATP synthase complex V at concentrations of 30-100 nM [33]. Cells with oxidative phenotype, was more likely to be inhibited. Cancer cells can shift their mechanism of ATP production from oxidative phosphorylation to Aerobic glycolysis as nutrients become depleted, causing cell death.

4.4 Mollecarbamates

Mollecarbamates A-D po repeating O-carboxyphenethylamide units and a carbamate moiety. Molleures B-E contains tetra- and penta- repeating carboxyphenethylamide units and a urea bridge in different positions and molledihydroisoquinolone, a cyclic form of O-Carboxyphenethylamide. These metabolites were found to be the only compound known to contain Ortho-carboxyphenethylamide derivatives in their skeleton. None of these compounds produced any antibacterial or antiviral properties [34].

4.5 Palmirolide A

A macrocyclic polyketide isolated from the ascidian *Synoicum adareanum.* Palmirolide A displays selective cytotoxicity towards melanoma by inhibiting V-ATPase [35].

4.6 Phosphoeleganin

A novel phosphorylated polyketide isolated from ascidian *Sidnyum elegans* [36]. It has no sufficient cytotoxic activity against human prostate cancer cells and human breast cancer cell. It subsequently inhibits the activity of Protein tyrosine phosphatase 1B [37].

5. Polyketides from ascidian associated microbes

5.1 Patellazoles

Patellazoles A-C (**Figure 3**) are a family of compounds produced by the alpha-proteobacterium *Candidatus Endolissoclinum faulkneri*, a microbe found in association with the ascidian *Lissoclinum Patella*. It shows cytotoxicity towards HCT 116 cells by inhibiting protein synthesis. It has several functional roles such as arresting of cell cycle at G1/S phases, and induces cell apoptosis [38].

5.2 Cyanobactins biosynthesis

Cyanobactin gene clusters are capable of encoding, two protease genes, A(N-terminal) and G(C-terminal) that are related to patA and patG genes from the patellamide biosynthetic pathway. A precursor peptide gene E being an homolog to patE which directly encodes cyanobactin structure that acts as a substrate for post translational modifications. Cyanobactin gene clusters may also encode homologs of PatD or PatF, denoted as D-protein and F-protein. Includes thiazoline/oxazoline dehydrogenases (responsible for the aromatization of the heterocycles to thiazoles and oxazoles, methyltransferases. This gene was proven to be essential for the synthesis of non-prenylated patellamides. Cyanobactins are classified into different groups based on a correspondence between genotypes and chemotypes.

5.2.1 Biosynthetic pathway

Cyanobactin biosynthesis begins with the precursor E-peptide, which is composed of an N-terminal conserved leader sequence that is recognized by some of the modifying and cleaving enzymes. Cyanobactin genetic cluster may also employ more than one precursor peptide. Genetic cluster may contain upto10 precursor peptide gene. E-peptide that contains the enzyme recognition sequences, 1,4 hypervariable core regions may be present and dictate amino acid backbone of cyanobactins.

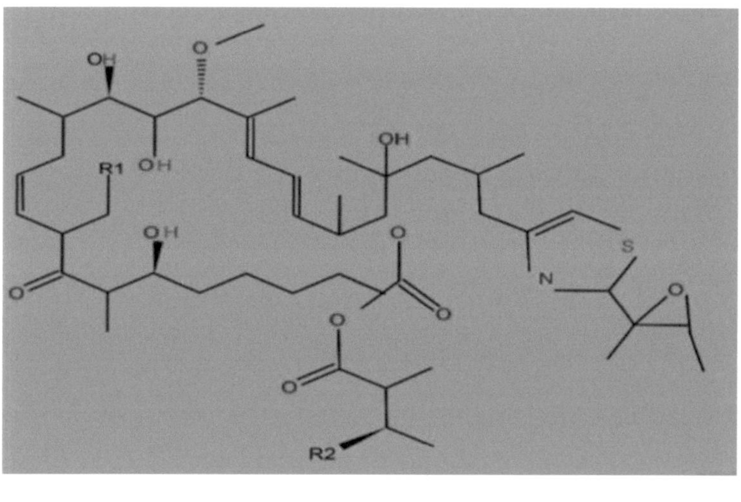

Figure 3.
Structures of Patellazoles A–C [31]. Adapted from Kwan and Schmidt.

Cyanobactins are ribosomally synthesized and post-translationally modifies peptides produced in the ribosome. Biosynthetic enzymes for cyclic peptide synthesis are encoded in the *Prochloron* genome. Precursor peptides are post-translationally modified by various enzymes adding the heterocycles derived from the cysteine, serine and threonine or isoprene units. Modifies peptides are cleaved from the precursor and cyclized to the natural products [39]. These products are capable of exhibiting combinatorial biosynthesis. Ribosomally synthesized and post translationally modified peptides combinatorial chemistry is made mainly because of the core peptide hypervariably, broad substrate [40] specificity, enzyme recognition sequences and modularity of post-translational elements. Many of these post-translational modifications are found in marine organisms. Mechanisms as well as the gene cluster involved in the formation of the thiazoline and oxazoline rings in cyanobactin are well studied. Patellamide pathway, coded by the pat gene cluster which is commomly expressed in *Prochloron* involves several enzymatic steps: Aminoacid heterocyclization, cleavage, peptide cleavage, peptide macrocyclization, heterocycle oxidation and epimerization. Some of the closely related products are also prenylated (**Figure 4(a, b)**).

In the presence of D-protein cyclodehydratase, heterocyclization of cysteins, serines or threonines will be directed by sequence recognition. A protease cleaves the precursor peptide RSII, leaving a free amine available for macrocyclization. G-protease splits the precursor peptide RSIII and causes the catalization of C-N macrocyclization. Other transformations may occur such as, prenylation of serine/threonines and tyrosines/tryptophans residues catalyzed by the PatF class of prenyltransferases. Oxidation of heterocycles to oxazoles and thiazoles when oxidized, domain is present within the G gene or separate and geranylation [41].

5.2.2 Heterocyclase

Heterocyclase accompanies heterocyclization of cysteins, serine and threonine residues to thiazolines or oxazolines and eliminates water. Cyanobactins heterocyclases D has been studied in partellamide and trunkamide pathways. Heterocyclases D in both pathways is ATP dependent. An adenylase mechanism has been proposed for TruD, from trunkamide.

An adenylase mechanism has been proposed for TruD, from trunkamide pathway, whose crystal structure presents as the three, domain protein. Enzyme progreesivity requires the presence of a lead protein to be attached to the core, indicating that heterocyclization occurs before cleavage and macrocyclization of the precursor peptide.

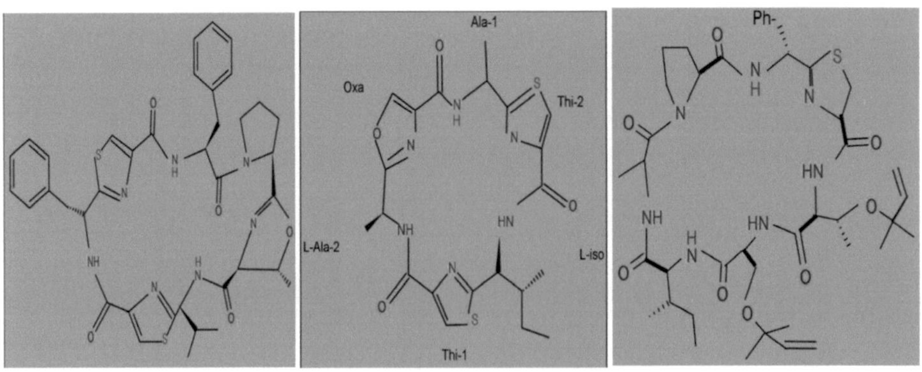

a) b) c)

Figure 4.
a)bistratamide M, b) bistratamide N produced from c) Trunkamide A.

The sequence element present in the lead sequence is responsible for heterocyclization. Cyanobactin pathway encoding a heterocyclase modifies a oxidase domain responsible for oxidation of thiazolines and oxazoles to thiazoles and oxazoles.

5.2.3 Macrocyclization

PatA protease from patellamide gene cluster catalyzes the N-terminal protease cleavage from the precursor peptide removing the leader sequence. This reaction catalyzed by the N-terminal protease A and C-terminal protease G, under subtilisin protein family encoded by cyanobactin gene cluster. A kind of protease called PatG isolated from Prochlorom was found to macrocyclize a wide range of synthetic substrates with non-proteinogenic and D-amino acids. Macrocyclase consists of PatG and PagG structural domains representing a catalytic triad. Macrocyclase crystal structure represents a domain of PatG, showing subtilisin folds containing two helices presented by the macrocyclization insert without any change in sequence length. This domain is insensitive to the identity of the residues within the core peptides, as PatG acts on RSIII residues and catalyzes the C-N macrocyclization. During this process, PatA protease removes the amino terminal linked to the core, producing a free amino terminal and PatG protease removes a catalytic terminal flanking the core. Cleaving site is protected by the PatG protease preventing access to water and continues hydrolysis until the transduction reactiobn is completed. PatG emphasizes macrocyclic peptide formation, by removing the C-terminal protease.

5.2.4 Prenylation

Prenylagarmide (pag), trunkamide (tru). Aesturamide (lyn) pathways, encodes the prenyltransferase gene, capable of synthesizing prenylated compounds. Prenyltransferase gene present in patellamide, generates non-prenylated patellamide A and C. Trunkamide contains O-prenylated threonine and serine (**Figure 4(c)**). Prenylagarmide contains O-prenylated tyrosine. Prenyltransferase from lyn (LynF) and tru (TruF) pathways. Prenyltransferase from lyn (LynF) and tru (TruF) pathways have been characterized biochemically. However, the reverse O-Prenylated tyrosine undergoes spontaneous claisen rearranging and yieding ortho-substituited phenol. LynF prenylates the oxygen atom of tyrosine residue by using dimethylallylpyrophosphate (DMAPP). TruF prenylates serine and threonine residues on the hydroxyl side chain. PatF from the patellamide pathway, it embraces the other prenyltransferase, classic TIM barrel fold. No enzymatic activity was detected, may be due to absence of prenylation in patellamides A and C. PatF essential for the production of patellamide in vivo and consequently responsible for another function in this pathway. Oxidase domain is conserved among PatG homologs and studies put up a prediction that FMN id dependent. Thiazoline oxidase has been related in sequence to the patellamide enzyme. However its action on microcin pathway was a matter of biochemical study. How this enzyme recognizes the substrate remains unclear, as the microns are linear and patellamides are macrocyclase. One homolog of the oxidase domain of PatG was capable of oxidizing both linear and macrocycle thiazoline containing compounds and another homolog has the ability to perform oxidation on a macrocyclic substrate.

5.2.5 DUF

PatA and PatG proteases contain a domain of unknown function sharing a sequence similarity of about 56%. DUF domains are found in PatA and PatG from the patellamide biosynthetic clusters. Epimerization follows heterocyclization and precedes oxidation. Epimerization is an important role of DUF domain, and its phenomenon is chemically spontaneous. Crystal structure of PatG-DUF is a novel fold dimer with two zinc ions. Practical importance of the dimer remains unclear since, the residues involved in Zn2+ binding, which is necessary for dimerization are not conserved among DUF domains. DUF domain does not bind to the macrocycle or the core peptide alone.

6. Sulfer containing metabolites

6.1 Polysulfides and alkylsulfides

Sulfur atom rarely found among the marine organism. Ascidians belonging to the genus *Lissoclinum (didemnidae)* had shown resistant towards Plasmodium chemical scaffolds, some of them with unique antiviral activity against mammalian erythrocytes. Among these metabolites, several structurally intriguing antimicrobial polysulfides have activity comparable to the commercially available antimalarials chloroquine and quinine shows activity against bacteria, fungi and other infective agents. Antifungal properties of benzopentathiepin varacin isolated from *L.perforatum*. Due to its antifungal properties, they paved the way for the isolation of.

Lissoclinotoxins A and B. Toxins isolated from *L.vareau* showed activity against *Candida albicans* with a 14 mm zone of inhibition. Polysufides showed an activity of strong cytotoxicity, being 100times more potent than 5 against *Staphylococcus aureus.* Having a minimum inhibitory concentration IC90 of 0.05ug/ml against human colon cancer HCT 116. Role of ascidian associated microorganism, showed activity against *Aeromonas salmonicida* and *Vibrio anguillarium*. Role played by the ascidian associated microorganism in the synthesis and cytotoxic activity was tested against the *Aeromonas salmonicida* and *Vibrio anguillarium* by the zonal inhibition assays of their secondary metabolites reported by the discovery of analogues lissoclinotoxin B. It is a potent inhibitor of bacteria, mainly against the *Aeromonas salmonicidia*. Varacin isolated from the colonial ascidian exhibited antimicrobial properties. It had moderate cytotoxic effects against the Polycitor species. Varacin showed active resistance towards the strain Plasmodium isolated and also exhibited strong activity in vitro against the *Candida albicans*. On the other hand, this peptide exhibited a lower IC 50 value at 296 nM towards the Gram-positive *Bacillus subtilis* [42]. Further, three polysulfites isolated from the colonial ascidian, was isolated as acetates, 4-Trichosporon metagrophytes and it showed resistance to *Candida albicans* with an MIC of 20 and 40 μg/mL.

6.2 Bengacarboline

A beta-carboline alkaloid derived from the ascidian *Didemnin* species, known to contain cytotoxic effect on in vitro A26 human tumor cell line and inhibit topoisomerase II activity [43].

6.3 Ihenyamines A-B

A derivative from the ascidian, *Polycitorella* species containing compounds exhibiting moderate cytotoxicity towards in-vitro cell line studies. Alkaloids of *Staurosporine*, studied on the MONO-MAC-6 cell lines, successfully inhibited the cancer growth and are known to be strong inhibitors of Protein kinase [44]. Pibocin B isolated from the Japan ascidian *Eudistoma* species, has a unique strucrtural species of N-O methylindole alkaloid and known to produce moderate cytotoxic [45] (Makarieva et al.,) effect towards mouse *Ehrlich* carcinoma cells with an ED50 25 μg/mL (**Figure 5**).

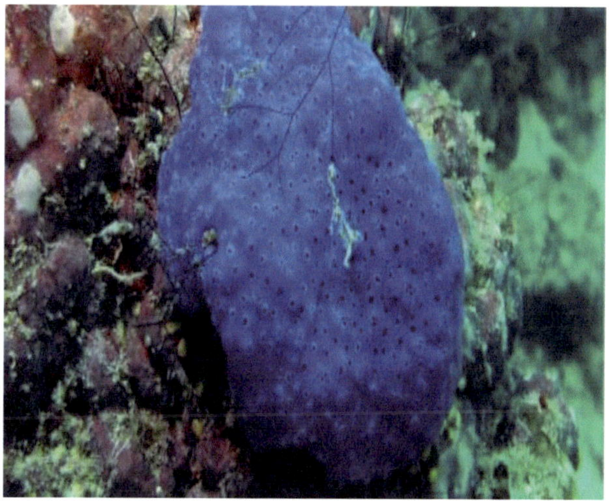

Figure 5.
Showing image of ascidian Eudistoma *species.*

6.4 Shishijimicins A-C

A class of beta-carboline alkaloids, isolated from the ascidian *Didemnum proliferum*. These peptides are potent antitumorigenic agents [46]. Three classes of alkaloids isolated from the Guinea sea squirt *Eudistoma* species consists of Rigidin, RigidinE and 1-methylherbiproline. These three alkaloids were reported to contain moderate inhibitory potential towards human P53 colon carcinoma cell lines and A431 epidermal carcinoma cell lines [47].

An alkaloid Fascaplysin isolated from the sponge *Fascaplysinopsis Bergquist* species, contained an excellent cytotoxic activity against murine C38 CFU cell lines and human H116 cell lines [48]. Meridianins, are brominated 3-(2-aminopyrimidine)-indole alkaloids isolated from the ascidian *Aplidium meridianum*. It is shown to have anti-proliferative effects, inducing apoptosis and inhibiting various cyclin dependent protein kinases, casein kinase-1 and glycogen synthase kinase-3 in NT2 teratocarcinoma cells [49].

6.5 Lamellarin D

This alkaloid represents an excellent cytotoxic effects towards tumor cells and proposed to be an anticancer agent for targeted topoisomerase –I cancer therapy [50]. This series of alkaloids represents an ideal source for developing anti-cancer agents. A few aspects of the various mechanism imposed by the lamellarin analogue, made this peptide to be used in biotechnology and pharmaceutical industries [51] (Marco et al.,).

Schupp and his co-workers reported alkaloids of Staurosporine and their eight subderivative alkaloids analogues such as 3-hydroxystaurosporine, 4-N-demethylstaurosporine, 3-demethoxy-3-hydroxylstaurosporine, 3-hydroxy-3-demethoxy-3-hydroxystaurosporine, 11-hydroy-4-N-demethylstaurosporine, 11-hydroxystaurosporine, 4-N-methylstaurosporine, 3-hydroxystaurosporine. These alkaloids were isolated from *Eudistoma toealensis*, a colonial ascidian and its alkaloids are being used in biotechnology and pharmaceutical industries.

6.6 Somocystinamide A

A lipopeptide isolated from *Lyngbya majuscula* (**Figure 6**), showed potent cytotoxic activity against N2A cells. It was found to be an potent apoptosis inducer

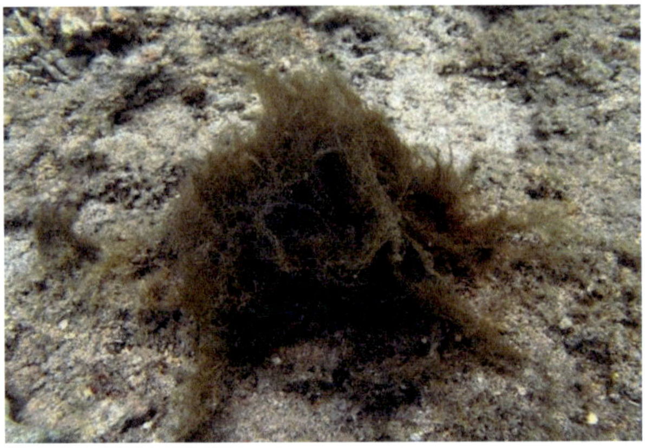

Figure 6.
Image showing ascidian Lyngbya majuscula.

towards a number of cell lines, activation of caspase 8 and angiogenic endothelial cells via intrinsic and extrinsic pathways.

6.7 Apratoxin A

A cyclodepsipeptide isolated from ascidian, *Lyngbya majuscula* showed antiproliferative activity in KB and LoVo cancer cells. It induces the antiproliferative activity through the induction of G1 cell cycle arrest, apoptotic cascade and partially initiated by antagonism of FGF signaling via STAT3 [52].

7. Cyanobacteria

Cyanobacteria, known as blue-green algae, are ancient photosynthetic prokaryotes which inhabit a wide diversity of habitats including tropical reefs, fresh water ponds, streams and puddles and fresh water ponds. Luxuriant growth of cyanobacteria in these adverse environments conditions is based on their abilities of forming resistant spores, opportunistically colonizing micro-habitants and surviving under conditions of high UV-flux through production of UV-absorbing pigments, has made them one of the successful life forms on earth. Cyanobacteria associated with ascidians, their symbotic relationship was first found out in 1982 by Kott.

Cyanobacteria are phylum of bacteria that produce oxygen during photosynthesis. Host ascidians that exhibit symbiotic relationship with cyanobacteria, Prochloron, which belong to the Didemidae family and are therefore called as "Didemnin ascidians". Cyanobacterial symbionts can both provide nutrients by means of Carbon fixation, nitrogen recycling and metabolite production and also exhibits defensive reaction for the host ascidian. Ascidian host are capable of producing some of the nitrogen containing nutrients that are needed for the cyanobacterial symbionts growth and also protection against the ultra violet radiation. Additional feature is that, a rich source of biologically active products, has assisted some of these organism to survive in predator-rich tropical reef ecosystems. Tropical marine Cyanobacteria particularly the filamentous forms such as *Lyngbya* species or *Symploca* species have been a source of novel natural products with therapeutic and biotechnological potential. Marine cyanobacteria are considered to be an important source of structurally diverse and biologically active natural products. Different peptides isolated from a wide variety of marine cyanobacteria, induces anticancer effects on various human cell lines. Most studied cytotoxic cyanobacteria on human tumor cell lines inducing minimal inhibitory effects [53].

Cyanobateria have a rich complement of photosynthetic pigments, including chlorophyll a and b, as well as several accessory pigments (phycoerythrin, phycocyanin, and allophycocyanin). Phycoerythrin has found application in biotechnology as a conjugate to antibiotics that then allow visualization of cellular constituents and processes and chlorophyll is being explored for its cancer chemotherapeutic activity. Apratoxin A is a cyclic depsipeptide extracted from *Lyngbya majuscule*. Exhibited cytotoxic effects on Human HeLa cervical carcinoma cells by cell cycle inhibition [54]. Similar mechanism was also reported on cyclic depsipeptide Coibamide A, isolated from *Leptolyngbya* species on Human lung cancer cell line and Lyngbyabellin B isolated from *Lyngbya majuscule* on Human Burkitt [55] lymphoma cells. Dolastatin 10 and Symplostatin 1, isolated from *Symploca* species, showed cytotoxic effect on human lung cancer cell line and Human breast carcinoma cell line by both Bcl-2 phosphorylation and Caspase-3 protein activation. Anticancer peptides such as *Lyngbya sp* and *Nostoc sp*, shows activity against cancer on different cell lines through microfilament disruption, secretory pathway inhibition.

Cyanobacteria inhibit Gram-negative and Gram-positive pathogenic bacterial species. Extracts of *Cylindrospermopsis raciborskii*, CYP011K and *Nostoc* species,

CENA69 possibly caused cancer cell inhibition. Extracts from *Fischerella* species, CENA213 showed inhibition of 3LL lung cancer cells. NPLJ-4 extracts isolated from *M.aeruginosa* reported to have inhibition against CT26 colon cancer cells. All of these extracts are prone to have low inhibitory activity towards human peripheral blood lymphocytes.

Aphanazomenon flos-aquae, freshwater cyanobacteria reported to contain immune stimulating properties, Other cyanobacteria Spirulina, a rich source of digestable proteins with a complete complement of essential amino acids [56].

Lyngbya majuscule from Curacao, yielded metabolites with broad biological properties, including those with toxicity to arthropods, those toxic to fish and those toxic to gastropods.

Bisanthrantaquinones, isolated from blue green algae associated with the colonial ascidian *Ecteinascidia turbinate*. These are the antimicrobial metabolites from ascidian-associated cyanobacteria (**Figure** 7), available to date. It has greater antibacterial effectiveness, and has resistance towards multi-drug resistant bacteria and vancomycin-resistant *Enterococcus faecalis* with an MIC of 0.6 and 12uM [57].

Cyanobacteria are considered to be an important source of bioactive metabolites, with various aspects of cytotoxic, antiviral, anticancer, antimitotic, antimicrobial, specific enzyme inhibitor and immunosuppressive activity. Cyanobacteria holds the presence of non-ribosomal peptide synthetase and polyketide synthetase genes, owing it to be the potential for finding novel natural drug products from these organism. Thus, cyanobacterium species are a rich strain enriched with the source of natural products with potential for pharmacological and biotechnological applications.

7.1 Tubulin binding proteins

Microtubules play many significant roles in cell biology. Formation of microtubules results from the polymerization of the subunit protein tubulin, first into heterodimers subsequently binds end to end with other heterodimer forming a protofilament, which in turn interacts to form sheets and eventually microtubules. Specifically, assembly and motility are crucially for the formation of the spindle apparatus during cell replication and mitosis where microtubule fibers direct the separation of sister chromatids into the resulting daughter cells. In case of rapidly

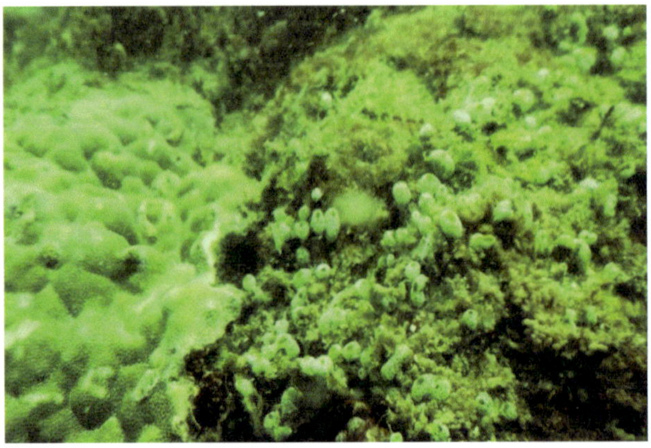

Figure 7.
Image showing marine cyanobacteria.

dividing cancer cells, microtubule assembly has been an important target in the development of new chemotherapeutic agents. Various drugs have developed to disrupt the process of mitosis and cause catastrophic cell death by either stabilizing microtubule complexes, caused by taxol. Depolymerization of the tubulin protein complex caused by Vinblastin [58]. Recently antimicrobial peptides targeting intracellular tubulin has developed from marine natural products.

Pharmacological properties of the marine mollusk, derivatives of *Aplysiidae* commonly know as the 'sea hare' or 'nudibrunch' has been reported for their toxic secretions. Biological activity of the cyanobacteria present in sea hare *Dolabella auricularia*, its structure consists of an active constituent, dolastatin 10. Dolastatin 10 displayed exceptional activity against the P388 lymphocytic leukemia cell line with ED50 value of about 4.6*10-5 g/ml. It is also reported to have potent antineoplastic activity. Dolastatin 10 isolated from field collections of the marine cyanobacterim *Symploca* species, clarifying the concept that the true biosynthetic source is the cyanobacteria and not the sea hare. Dolastatin 10, a unique linear pentapeptide is composed of four novel amino acid residues such as dolavaline, dolaisoleucine, dolaproline, dolaphenine and valine. High resolution mass spectroscopic analysis such as 1H (COSY, 2D-J resolved) and 13C NMR methodologies revealed the structure of this linear pentapeptide. This peptide sequence was assigned on the basis of several low resolution mass spectral fragmentation techniques. This peptide was found to be involved in the binding of Dolastatin 10, whereas other antimicrobial peptides near the exchangeable nucleotide and vinca alkaloid sites on microtubules [59]. Dolastatin 10 inhibits microtubule assembly in vitro and subsequently blocks cytokinesis. Also this peptide was noted for its non-competitive inhibition of radiolabeled vinblastine and vincristine to tubulin as well as tubulin dependent hydrolysis of GTP.

Dolastatin 10 binds to the 'peptide groove' lying within the r- subunit of tubulin. Molecular modeling suggested that the chiral centers of dolavaline, valine and dolaisoleucine binds in a manner that require the dolaphenine moiety to sterically block access to the vinca alkaloid and exchangeable nucleotide binding sites. Evidence of noncompetitive inhibition of Vinca alkaloid binding was realized by observation that tubulin polymerization and nucleotide binding are substantially diminished at sub-stoichiometric concentrations of dolastatin 10.

Dolastatin 10, on its Phase II clinical trial proved to be an antitumor agent, by evaluating its antitumor efficacy in patients with measurable recurrences of platinum –sensitive ovarian carcinoma in relation to the degree of toxicity [60].

7.2 Dolastatin 15

Dolabella auricularia, cyanobacteria associated sea hare contained another cytotoxic peptide called as dolastatin 15 (**Figure 8**). It was discovered by the process of bioassays guided fractionation and purified it as a minor fraction of about 6.2 mg from 1600 kg of wet sea hare. It was evident that this compound is well associated with the sea hare from its cyanobacterial diet. Dolastatin 15 is a linear heptadepsi-peptide composed of the dolavaline (N,N- dimethyl valine), valine, N-Me-valine, proline (x2), 2-hydroxyisovaleric acid. New Dpy moiety present in this peptide was proposed to be originated biosynthetically from the N-acetyl-phenyalanine methyl ester by intramolecular condensation. This peptide showed specific activity towards the P388 lymphocyte leukemia cell line of the national cancer institute (NCI) [61]. Dolastatin 15 was found to bind in the Vinca alkaloid domain of the tubulin complex, a definitive binding site was not identified. On the other hand, this peptide was shown to weakly bind tubulin with concurrent weak inhibition of crytptophyccin 1 binding, its specific acts are still unclear. Further on going work could determine the molecular mechanism of dolastatin 15 activity, although it has been stopped to enter the preclinical trials due to its general toxicity.

7.3 Actin binding proteins

Actin cytoskeleton is a dynamic network of filaments, which is associated with several proteins, plays an important role in cell shape, motility and signal transduction, this further switches on the other processes like embryonic development, tissue repair, immune response and tumor formation. However in cancer biology, actin cytoskeleton and actin associated proteins undergo modification in transformed tumor cell and impose ability to adhere and metastasize. It can be used for developing new chemotherapeutic agents. Actin targeting molecules could disrupt actin by destabilizing the filaments or induce hyperpolymerization [62].

7.4 Hectochlorin

Marine cyanobacteria *Lyngbya majuscula* provided a suitable source for the isolation of Hectochlorin. It was a potent antifungal agent. It showed activity towards

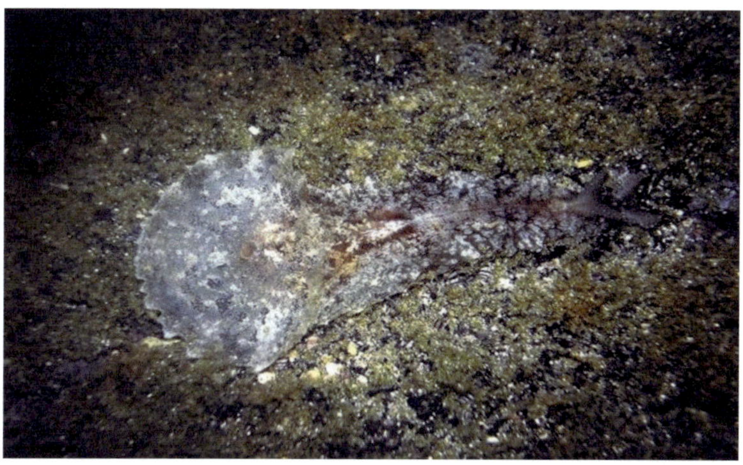

Figure 8.
Image showing Dolabella auricularia.

the Ptk2 cells derived from *Potorous tridactylus*, when treated with hectochlorin showed an increase in the number of the binucleated cells as a result of arresting the cytokinesis process. This peptide is very similar in action to jasplakinolode, in promoting hyperpolymerization of actin. Main difference that lies in between hectochlorin and jasplakinolode is that former can displace fluorescently labeled phalloidin from actin polymers, while the latter have two distinct interactions with actin. Hectochlorin, also strong potential towards the cell lines in the colon, melanoma, ovarian and renal sub-panels [63]. It showed a flat response curve against most cell lines, a specific activity of the compounds that are anti-proliferative but not directly cytotoxic [60].

7.5 Lyngbyabellins

This specific peptide was isolated from *Lyngbya majuscula* from south pacific and Caribbean and bear suitable structural resemblances to hectochlorin and dolabellin. Structural of lyngbyabellin A was determined using 2D NMR techniques and its absolute stereochemistry was determined by the chiral HPLC analysis. Lyngbyabellin A exhibited IC50 value of 0.03 μg/mL and 0.50 μg/mL against KB cells (human nasopharyngeal carcinoma cell line) and LoVo cells (human colon adenocarcinoma cells). It also disrupt the microfilament network in fibroblastic A10 cells at 0.01–5.0 μg/mL [64]. At higher concentrations of Lyngbyabellin A many cells became binucleate, an observation which inhibits cytokinesis. Lyngbyabellin B was found to be less toxic than lyngbyabellin A with IC 50 value of 0.10 μg/mL. It produces the same effects as hectochlorin on PtK2 cells, increase in number of binucleate cells were observed, when 10 M of the agent was treated with the cells. This finding proposed that actin is the main cellular target of the lyngbyabellins.

8. Neurotoxic compounds

8.1 Antillatoxin

Lyngbya majuscula served as the source for the extraction of the crude extract of Curacao, found to be highly ichthyotoxic and molluscicidal. This extract was then fractionation and subsequent purification led to the finding of the potent lipopeptide ichthyotoxin, antillatoxin. Antillatoxin is one of the most ichthyotoxic metabolites isolated from a marine cyanobacterium with an LD50 value of 0.05 g/mL. Pharmacological studies showed that the antillatoxin was neurotoxic and rapidly morphologically changes in rat cerebellar granule neurons (CGC's), also includes bebling of neurite membranes. Toxic effects of Antillatoxin was remarkably reduced, when the cells were treated with NMDA receptor antagonists like dextrophan [65]. Thus, its toxic effects were mediating by NMDA receptor dependent mechanism. Antillatoxin shown to be a powerful activator of voltage gated sodium channels and resembled brevetoxin. Unique biological activity of antillatoxin was mainly combined with its structure [66].

8.2 Antillatoxin

A lipopeptide isolated from *Lyngbya majuscula*, which is closely related to the antillatoxin with a larger B-methyl homophenylalanine instead of N-methyl valine residues was termed as Antillatoxin B. It is collectively found to be similar to ichthyotoxic (LC 50 = 1.0 M) and a potent activator of voltage gated sodium channels in mouse neuroblastoma cells [67].

8.3 Cyanobacterial metabolites

8.3.1 Barmamide

Isolated from the lipid extract of *Lyngbya majuscula* and consists of specific elements such as trichloromethyl group. Bioassays predicted that barbamide possesing anti-molluscicidal activity (LC 50 = 10.0 µg/mL) [68]. Whereas was found to be inactive in other assays and its biological properties still remains unknown.

8.3.2 Botryllus schlosseri

A specific bacterial species associated with *Botryllus schlosseri* was isolated and tested for their specific biological activities. *Bortyllus schlosseri* is a colonial ascidian composed of several tiny individual zooids enveloped by single tunic. Its an native to Europe. MTT analysis performed confirmed the cytotoxic activity of the crude extracts of the isolated bacterial strains. Extracts showed that, about 90% of the extracts showed cytotoxicity towards human heptatocellular carcinoma Bcl 7402 cells and human cervical carcinoma cell lines HeLa. Antimicrobial activity of the ascidian *Botryllus schlosseri* associated bacterial extracts showed that, it inhibits Gram-negative bacteria, Gram-positive bacteria, human pathogenic fungi and aquatic animal pathogenic bacteria. Thus, it exhibited higher incidence of resistance towards Gram-positive bacteria such as *Bacillus subtilis* and *Staphylococcus aureus* than Gram-negative bacteria [69].

9. Symbiotic organisms

Symbiotic bacteria contribute secondary metabolites necessary for defense and the survival of ascidians. About 80 percent of the currently available secondary metabolites obtained from ascidians were made only by its symbiotic bacteria. These metabolites are essential for the interaction between the host and symbiont and the bacteria are phylogenetically diverse [70].

9.1 Callynormine A

This peptide represents a new class of heterodetic cyclic peptides possessing an –amido-aminoacrylamide cyclization functionality. Cyclic endiamino peptides composed of a Hyp part [71], which is likely to be present in its peptides such as callynormine A and callyaerin A-D.

9.2 Gombamide A

A cyclothiopeptide consisting of an unusual amino acid residues like pHSA and pyroGlu [72]. It possess moderate inhibitory action towards the, Na^+/K^+-ATPase.

A specific new class of proline rich cycloheptapeptides derived from the photooxidation of tryptophan consisting of cytotoxic phakellistatin 3 and isophakellistatin 3. This peptides has an unusual amino acid residue such as “Hpi” respectively. These proline rich peptides act in a very divergent way, capable of causing stereospecific interaction with the membrane system. These interactions are caused by the intracellular targeting, compared to the general membrane disruption mode of action of the conventional antimicrobial peptides. It was found that proline rich antimicrobial peptides stereo specifically binds the intracellular foreign particles, such as the bacterial heat shock proteins DnaK. These peptides have a good water solubility, high potential for killing bacteria and lower cytotoxic activity at higher concentrations, these factors contribute to the development of the novel antimicrobial therapeutic agents in the field of medicine [73].

These peptides could easily enter the bacterial cell, binding and disrupting specific targets such as ribosome, thereby inhibiting protein synthesis. However all these factors, concludes that these peptides could subsequently be used as molecular hooks, for identifying intracellular or membrane proteins involved in this mechanism of action [74]. And it could be used for specifically altering novel therapeutics for drug delivery.

Scleritodermin A causes inhibition of tubulin polymerization [75].

Immunosuppressive activity of cyclolinopeptide A results from the formation of complex with cyclophilin and causing inhibition of phosphatase activity of calcineurin, plays an important role in T-lymphocyte signaling [76].

Cemadotin, a water soluble synthetic component of linear peptide dolastatin 15, which is reported to act on microtubules and causing strong suppression of microtubule dynamics [77].

9.3 Didemnin B

A cyclic depsipeptide derived from the marine cyclopolypeptide undergo clinical trials because of its potential to target oncological patients. Its high toxicity, poor solubility and shorter life span led to the discontinuation of didemnin B in clinical trials [78].

Didemnin B, belonging to a class of heterodetic non-polar cyclic peptide associated with several Antiviral, antitumor, immunomodulating properties, potency inhibits protein and DNA synthesis by binding to eukaryotic translation elongation factor EF-1 in a GTP dependent manner. Formation of the [79] Didemnin B-GTP-EF-1 complex could be responsible for protein synthesis inhibition.

Inhibition of protein synthesis by didemnin B occurs by stabilization of aminoacyl-tRNA to the ribosomal A-site, preventing the translocation of phenylalanyl–tRNA from the A- to the P-site, preventing peptide bond formation.

Tamandarin A acts in a very same mechanism as didemnin B. Aplidine's involves several mechanism of action such as cell cycle arrest and protein synthesis inhibition. It induces early oxidative stress and results in a rapid activation of JNK and p38 MAPK phosphorylation by activating both kinases occurring among before the activation of apoptosis [80].

Didemnin B causes the death of several transformed cells through apoptosis, DNA fragmentation within the cytosol and generation of DNA ladders [81].

A linear depsipeptide kahalalide F, has predominant antifungal and antitumor activity, and underway in clinical trials.

A cyclic depsipeptide Plitidepsin (dehydrodedemnin B or aplidine) is in its clinical trial for being developing it as a drug. In 2003, plitidepsin was given orphan drug status for treating acute lymphoblastic leukemia. In 2007, it underwent phase II clinical trials and in 2006 it is announced for small phase-I clinical trials for treating multiple myeloma [82].

Antimitotic dolastatins group, dolastatin 10 and 15 are undergoing phase-II clinical trials. A synthetic analogue of dolastatin 15, cemadotin is also in phase-II clinical trials for its promising cancer chemotherapeutic agent.

9.4 Ecteinascidian—743

A specific alkaloid isolated from the tunicate *Ecteinascidia turbinate*, represents a rich source of symbionts whose aqueous extract are known to contain anticancerous agents. Ecteinascidin alkaloids molecular structures are known to be defined as complex tetrahydroisoquinolones. This alkaloid is a major meatabolite possessing cytotoxic activity against leukemia cells (IC 50 0.5 ng/mL). Ecteinascidins structure is considered to be of a natural microbial origin (eg saframycins) [83]. This alkaloid because of its stability and relatively high natural abundance made it most suitable for entering clinical trials. Ecteinascidians-743, entered phase-I clinical trials after rendering, to have an higher therapeutic index and potency. Recently, it was found that ET-743binds to the minor groove of DNA to induce a bend in the DNA helix towards the major groove. ET-743 plays an important role in causing interference with the cellular transcription coupled nucleotide excision repair to induce cell death and cytotoxicity which is independent of p53 status. However, advanced ovarian, breast and mesenchymal tumors showed more response to ET-743 in phase-I clinical trials. ET-743 in phase-II clinical trials showed more heightened response towards soft tissue sarcoma (STS), ovarian and breast cancer. There are two patents for bacterial symbionts of the tunicate *Ecteinascidia turbinata*, primary focus was on the isolation of the producing microbe, secondary one uses 16S rDNA sequences to identify the endosymbiont as *Endoecteinascidia frumentensis*, the source for producing the ecteinascidins [84].

9.5 Helichondrin B

A complex polyether derived from the marine animals such as sponges, tunicates and their various predators. Compounds such as palytoxin, maitotoxin and halichondrins, because of their potential even very small quantities of these compounds could aid valuable commercial sense. Halichondrins was first isolated from the Japanese sponge *Halichondrin okadai* (Uemura). Halichondrin B and several natural analogs were subsequently been derived from various sponges such as, *Lissodendoryx* species, *Phakellia carteri* and *Axinella* species, thus it strongly suggest that this type may be constructed by an ascidian associated microorganism. A number of studies reported their cell toxicity, and it was found that halichondrins are tubulin inhibitors, noncompatitively binding to the vinca binding site and causing a charateristics G2-M cell cycle arrest by concomitant disruption of the mitotic spindle. *Dysidea herbacea*, a sponge and its symbiotic cyanobacterium *Oscillatoria spongellae*. These cyanobacterial cells are known to contain a series of highly distinctive chlorinated peptides, which has strong structural precedence in metabolites isolated from the free-living cyanobacterium *Lyngbya majusculea*. However a similar peptide from tunicate *Lissoclinum patella*, harbors an abundance of cyanobacterium *Prochloron* species which produces a series of distinctive cyclic peptides, associated with both cyanobacterial and tunicate cells. Palytoxin and maitotoxin are both available as research biochemicals [85].

9.6 C-Phycocyanin

A blue green pigment-protein complex isolated from the marine cyanobacteria *Agmenellum quadruplicatum, Mastigoclaudus laminosus*. This pigment appeared to be an activator of pro-apoptotic gene and also the down regulator of anti-apoptotic gene expressions [86]. Its activity of apoptosis on HeLa cell lines in-vitro, resulted from the transduction of apoptosis signals. These apoptosis further leads to the path of cell shrinkage, membrane bebbing, nuclear condensation and DNA fragment known to be observed from A549 and HT29 treated with C-phycocyanin.

10. Conclusion

However, a handful of antimicrobial peptides have found to be approved today for clinical use as anti-infectives. Cyclic peptides such as gramicidins and polymyxins are well characterized. Gramicidins are used in treating infections such as infection of the surface wounds as well as the infections of nasal, ocular and throat infections. On the other hand polymyxins are used for treating eye infections prior to local administration and for selective decontamination of the digestive tract and also for systemic infections caused by drug-resistant gram-negative pathogens. Daptomycin, a cyclic antimicrobial peptides in clinical practice to treat skin complications and skin-structure infections caused by Gram-positive bacteria mostly, *Staphylococcus aureus*. Omiganan, a 12 amino acid analog of indolicidin, has been incorporated in the local treatment of Catheter related infections, atopic dermatitis, genital warts, acne vulgaris. Pexiganan, a 22 amino acid analog being evaluated in the Phase III clinical trials for the treatment of mild diabetic foot ulcers, burns and decubitus ulcers. PXL01, iron-binding lactoferritin present in milk and mucosal secretions, evaluated in phase II clinical trials for treating post-operative adhesions in patients undergoing flexor tendon repair surgery of the hands [87].

Author details

Rajaian Pushpabai Rajesh* and Grace Vanathi M
Center for Nanomedical Sciences, Sathyabama Institute of Science and Technology, India

*Address all correspondence to: jeshran@gmail.com

References

[1] Berlinck RGS, Britton R, Piers E, Lim L, Roberge M, Rocha RM, Andersen RJ (1998) Granulatimide and isogranulatimide, aromatic alkaloids with G2 checkpoint inhibition activity iso- lated from the Brazilian ascidian Didemnum granulatum: structure elucidation and synthesis. J Org Chem 63:9850-9856.

[2] Bibby TS, Nield J, Chen M, Larkum AWD, Barber J (2003) Structure of a photosystem II supercomplex isolated from Prochloron didemni retaining its chlorophyll a/b light-har- vesting system. Proc Natl Acad Sci USA 100:9050-9054.

[3] Blunt JW, Copp BR, Munro MHG, Northcote PT, Princep MR (2005) Marine natural products. Nat Prod Rep 22:15-61 Britton R, de Oliveira JHHL, Andersen RJ, Berlinck RGS (2001).

[4] Granulatimide and 6-bromogranulatimide, minor alkaloids of the Brazilian ascidian Didemnum granulatum. J Nat Prod 64:254-255.

[5] Bugni TS, Ireland CM (2004) Marine-derived fungi: a chemically and biologically diverse group of microorganisms. Nat Prod Rep 21:143-163.

[6] Dunham P, Weissmann G (1986) Aggregation of marine sponge cells induced by Ca pulses, Ca ionophores, and phorbol es- ters proceeds in the absence of external Ca. Biochem Bio- phys Res Commun 134:1319-1326.

[7] Faulkner DJ (2002) Marine natural products. Nat Prod Rep 19:1– 48.

[8] Faulkner DJ, Newman DJ, Cragg GM (2004) Investigations of the marine Xora and fauna of the Islands of Palau. Nat Prod Rep 21:50-76.

[9] Groepler W, Schuett C (2003) Bacterial community in the tunic matrix of a colonial ascidian Diplosoma migrans. Helgoland Mar Res 57: 139-143.

[10] Hildebrand M, Waggoner LE, Lim GE, Sharp KH, Ridley CP, Haygood MG (2004) Approaches to identify, clone, and ex- press symbiont bioactive metabolite genes. Nat Prod Rep 21:122-142.

[11] Anand, T. P., Chellaram, C., Kuberan, G., & Archana, H. (2012). Bioactive peptides from marine sources: A review. Indian Journal of Innovations and Developments, 1, 61-64. Andavan, G. S., & Lemmens-Gruber, R. (2010).

[12] Cyclodepsipeptides from marine sponges: Natural agents for drug research. Marine Drugs, 8, 810-834. Aoki, S., Cao, L., Matsui, K., Rachmat, R., Akiyama, S. I., & Kobayashi, M. (2004).

[13] Kendarimide A, a novel peptide reversing P-glycoprotein-mediated multidrug resistance in tumor cells, from a marine sponge of Haliclona sp. Tetrahedron, 60, 7053-7059.

[14] Arai, M., Yamano, Y., Fujita, M., Setiawan, A., & Kobayashi, M. (2012). Stylissamide X, a new proline-rich cyclic octapeptide as an inhibitor of cell migration, from an Indonesian marine sponge of Stylissa sp. Bioorganic & Medicinal Chemistry Letters, 22, 1818-1821.

[15] Arnison, P. G., Bibb, M. J., Bierbaum, G., Bowers, A. A., Bugni, T. S., Bulaj, G., et al. (2013). Ribosomally synthesized and post-translationally modified peptide natural prod- ucts: Overview and recommendations for a universal nomenclature. Natural Product Reports, 30, 108-160.

[16] Asolkar, R. N., Freel, K. C., Jensen, P. R., Fenical, W., Kondratyuk, T. P., Park, E. J., et al. (2009). Arenamides

A-C, cytotoxic NFκB inhibitors from the marine actinomycete Salinispora arenicola. Journal of Natural Products, 72, 396-402.

[17] Won, T.H.; You, M.; Lee, S.H.; Rho, B.J.; Oh, D.C.; Oh, K.B.; Shin, J. Amino Alcohols from the Ascidian *Pseudodistoma* Sp. Mar. Drugs **2014**, *12*, 3754-3769.

[18] Kossuga, M.H.; MacMillan, J.B.; Rogers, E.W.; Molinski, T.F.; Nascimento, G.G.F.; Rocha, R.M.; Berlinck, R.G.S. (2S,3R)-2-Aminododecan-3-Ol, a New Antifungal Agent from the Ascidian *Clavelina Oblonga*. J. Nat. Prod. **2004**, *67*, 1879-1881.

[19] Wang, J.; Pearce, A.N.; Chan, S.T.S.; Taylor, R.B.; Page, M.J.; Valentin, A.; Bourguet-Kondracki, M.L.; Dalton, J.P.; Wiles, S.; Copp, B.R. Biologically Active Acetylenic Amino Alcohol and N-Hydroxylated 1,2,3,4-Tetrahydro-β-Carboline Constituents of the New Zealand Ascidian *Pseudodistoma Opacum*. J. Nat. Prod. **2016**, *79*, 607-610.

[20] Perron, F.; Albizati, K.F. Chemistry of Spiroketals. *Chem. Rev.* **1989**, *89*, 1617-1661.

[21] Aho, J.E.; Pihko, P.M.; Rissa, T.K. Nonanomeric Spiroketals in Natural Products: Structures, Sources, and Synthetic Strategies. Chem. Rev. **2005**, *105*, 4406-4440.

[22] Sperry, J.; Wilson, Z.E.; Rathwell, D.C.K.; Brimble, M.A. Isolation, Biological Activity and Synthesis of Benzannulated Spiroketalnatural Products. Nat. Prod. Rep. **2010**, *27*, 1117-1137.

[23] Zang, F.M.; Zhang, S.Y.; Tu, Y.Q. Recent Progress in the Isolation, Bioactivity, Biosynthesis, and Total Synthesis of Natural Spiroketals. Nat. Prod. Rep. **2018**, *35*, 75-104.

[24] Pika, J.; Faulkner, D.J. A Reinvestigation of the Didemnaketals from the Palauan Ascidian Didemnum Sp. Nat. Prod. Lett. **1995**, *7*, 291-296.

[25] Potts, B.C.M.; Faulkner, D.J. Didemnaketals A and B, HIV-1 Protease Inhibitors from the Ascidian Didemnum Sp. J. Am. Chem. Soc. **1991**, *113*, 6321-6322.

[26] Mohamed, G.A.; Ibrahim, S.R.M.; Badr, J.M.; Youssef, D.T.A. Didemnaketals D and E, Bioactive Terpenoids from a Red Sea Ascidian Didemnum Species. Tetrahedron **2014**, *70*, 35-40.

[27] Shaala, L.A.; Youssef, D.T.A.; Ibrahim, S.R.M.; Mohamed, G.A.; Badr, J.M.; Risinger, A.L.; Mooberry, S.L. Didemnaketals F and G, New Bioactive Spiroketals from a Red Sea Ascidian Didemnum Species. Mar. Drugs **2014**, *12*, 5021-5034.

[28] Cheung, R.C.; Ng, T.B.; Wong, J.H. Marine Peptides: Bioactivities and Applications. Mar. Drugs **2015**, *13*, 4006-4043.

[29] Kang, H.K.; Seo, C.H.; Park, Y. Marine Peptides and Their Anti-Infective Activities. Mar. Drugs **2015**, *13*, 618-654.

[30] Falanga, A.; Lombardi, L.; Franci, G.; Vitiello, M.; Iovene, M.R.; Morelli, G.; Galdiero, M.; Galdiero, S. Marine Antimicrobial Peptides: Nature Provides Templates for the Design of Novel Compounds against Pathogenic Bacteria. Int. J. Mol. Sci. **2016**, *17*, 785.

[31] Cruz, J.; Ortiz, C.; Guzman, F.; Fernandez-Lafuente, R.; Torres, R. Antimicrobial Peptides: Promising Compounds against Pathogenic Microorganisms. Curr. Med. Chem. **2014**, *21*, 2299-2321.

[32] Taylor, S.W.; Craig, A.G.; Fischer, W.H.; Park, M.; Lehrer, R.I. Styelin D,

an Extensively Modified Antimicrobial Peptide from Ascidian Hemocytes. J. Biol. Chem. **2000**, *275*, 38417-38426.

[33] Hurdle, J.G.; O'Neill, A.J.; Chopra, I.; Lee, R.E. Targeting Bacterial Membrane Function: An Underexploited Mechanism for Treating Persistent Infections. Nat. Rev. Microbiol. **2011**, *9*, 62-75.

[34] Lehrer, R.I.; Tincu, J.A.; Taylor, S.W.; Menzel, L.P.; Waring, A.J. Natural Peptide Antibiotics from Tunicates: Structures, Functions and Potential Uses. Integr. Comp. Biol. **2003**, *43*, 313-322.

[35] Lee, I.H.; Cho, Y.; Lehrer, R.I. Styelins, Broad-Spectrum Antimicrobial Peptides from the Solitary Tunicate, *Styela clava*. Comp. Biochem. Physiol. **1997**, *118B*, 515-521.

[36] Lee, I.H.; Zhao, C.; Cho, Y.; Harwig, S.S.L.; Cooper, E.L.; Lehrer, R.I. Clavanins, α-Helical Antimicrobial Peptides from Tunicate Hemocytes. FEBS Lett. **1997**, *400*, 158-162.

[37] Saude, A.C.; Ombredane, A.S.; Silva, O.N.; Barbosa, J.A.; Moreno, S.E.; Guerra Araujo, A.C.; Falcão, R.; Silva, L.P.; Dias, S.C.; Franco, O.L. Clavanin Bacterial Sepsis Control Using a Novel Methacrylate Nanocarrier. Int. J. Nanomed. **2014**, *9*, 5055-5069.

[38] Galinier, R.; Roger, E.; Sautiere, P.E.; Aumelas, A.; Banaigs, B.; Mitta, G. Halocyntin and Papillosin, Two New Antimicrobial Peptides Isolated from Hemocytes of the Solitary Tunicate, Halocynthia Papillosa. J. Pept. Sci. **2009**, *15*, 48-55.

[39] Lee, I.H.; Lee, Y.S.; Kim, C.H.; Kim, C.R.; Hong, T.; Menzel, L.; Boo, L.M.; Pohl, J.; Sherman, M.A.; Waring, A.; et al. Dicynthaurin: An Antimicrobial Peptide from Hemocytes of the Solitary Tunicate, *Halocynthia aurantium*. Biochim. Biophys. Acta **2001**, *1527*, 141-148.

[40] Jang, W.S.; Kim, K.N.; Lee, Y.S.; Nam, M.H.; Lee, I.H. Halocidin: A New Antimicrobial Peptide from Hemocytes of the Solitary Tunicate, *Halocynthia aurantium*. FEBS Lett. **2002**, *521*, 81-86.

[41] Jang, W.S.; Kim, H.K.; Lee, K.Y.; Kim, S.A.; Han, Y.S.; Lee, I.H. Antifungal Activity of Synthetic Peptide Derived from Halocidin, Antimicrobial Peptide from the Tunicate, *Halocynthia aurantium*. FEBS Lett. **2006**, *580*, 1490-1496.

[42] Jang, W.S.; Kim, C.H.; Kang, M.S.; Chae, H.J.; Son, S.M.; Seo, S.J.; Lee, I.H. CDNA Cloning of Halocidin and a New Antimicrobial Peptide Derived from the N-Terminus of Ci-META4. Peptides **2005**, *26*, 2360-2367.

[43] Hansen, I.K.Ø.; Isaksson, J.; Poth, A.G.; Hansen, K.Ø.; Andersen, A.J.C.; Richard, C.S.M.; Blencke, H.-M.; Stensvåg, K.; Craik, D.J.; Haug, T. Isolation and Characterization of Antimicrobial Peptides with Unusual Disulfide Connectivity from the Colonial Ascidian *Synoicum Turgens*. Mar. Drugs **2020**, *18*, 51.

[44] Oltz, E.M.; Bruening, R.C.; Smith, M.J.; Kustin, K.; Naganishi, K. The Tunichromes. A Class of Reducing Blood Pigments from Sea Squirts: Isolation, Structures, and Vanadium Chemistry. *J. Am.* Chem. Soc. **1988**, *110*, 6162-6172.

[45] Harrigan, G.G., Goetz, G.H., Luesch, H., Yang, S., Likos, J., 2001. Dysideaprolines A–F and barbaleucamides A–B, novel polychlorinated compounds from a Dysidea species. J. Nat. Prod. 64, 1133-1138.

[46] Horgen, F.D., Kazmierski, E.B., Westenburg, H.E., Yoshida, W.Y., Scheuer, P.J., 2002. Malevamide D: isolation and structure determi- nation

of an isodolastatin H analogue from the marine cyanobacte- rium Symploca hydnoides. J. Nat. Prod. 65, 487-491.

[47] Jordan, M.A., Wilson, L., 1998. Microtubules and actin filaments: dynamic targets for cancer chemotherapy. Curr. Opin. Cell Biol. 10, 123-130.

[48] Kimura, J., Takada, Y., Inayoshi, T., Nakao, Y., Goetz, G., Yoshida, W.Y., Scheuer, P.J., 2002. Kulokekahilide-1, a cytotoxic depsipeptide from the cephalaspidean mollusk Philinopsis speciosa. J. Org. Chem. 67, 1760-1767.

[49] Li, W.I., Berman, F.W., Okino, T., Yokokawa, F., Shioiri, T., Gerwick, W.H., Murray, T.F., 2001. Antillatoxin is a marine cyanobacterial toxin that potently activates voltage-gated sodium channels. Proc. Natl. Acad. Sci. USA 98, 7599-7604.

[50] Luesch, H., Pangilinan, R., Yoshida, W.Y., Moore, R.E., Paul, V.J., 2001a. Pitipeptolides A and B, new cyclodepsipeptides from the marine cyanobacterium Lyngbya majuscula. J. Nat. Prod. 64, 304-307.

[51] Luesch, H., Yoshida, W.Y., Moore, R.E., Paul, V.J., Corbett, T.H., 2001b. Total structure determination of apratoxin A, a potent novel cytotoxin from the marine cyanobacterium Lyngbya majuscula. J. Am. Chem. Soc. 123, 5418-5423.

[52] Luesch, H., Yoshida, W.Y., Moore, R.E., Paul, V.J., Mooberry, S.L., Corbett, T.H., 2002a. Symplostatin 3, a new dolastatin 10 analogue from the marine cyanobacterium Symploca sp. VP452. J. Nat. Prod. 65, 16-20.

[53] Luesch, H., Yoshida, W.Y., Moore, R.E., Paul, V.J., 2002b. Structurally diverse new alkaloids from Palauan collections of the apratoxin- producing marine cyanobacterium Lyngbya sp. Tetrahedron 58, 7959– 7966.

[54] Luesch, H., Harrigan, G.G., Goetz, G., Horgen, F.D., 2002c. The cyanobacterial origin of potent anticancer agents originally isolated from sea hares. Curr. Med. Chem. 9, 1791-1806.

[55] Luesch, H., Williams, P.G., Yoshida, W.Y., Moore, R.E., Paul, V.J., 2002d. Ulongamides A–F, new b-amino acid-containing cyclodepsi- peptides from Palauan collections of the marine cyanobacterium Lyngbya sp. J. Nat. Prod. 65, 996-1000.

[56] Luesch, H., Yoshida, W.Y., Moore, R.E., Paul, V.J., 2002e. New apratoxins of marine cyanobacterial origin from Guam and Palau. Bioorg. Med. Chem. 10, 1973-1978.

[57] Luesch, H., Chanda, S.K., Raya, R.M., DeJesus, P.D., Orth, A.P., Walker, J.R., Belmonte, J.C.I., Schultz, P.G., 2006. A functional genomic approach to the mode of action of apratoxin A. Nat. Chem. Biol. 2, 158-167.

[58] MacMillan, J., Ernst-Russell, M.A., de Ropp, J.S., Molinski, T.F., 2002. Lobocyclamides A–C, lipopeptides from a cryptic cyanobacterial mat containing Lyngbya confervoides. J. Org. Chem. 67, 8210-8215.

[59] Ma, D.-W., Zou, B., Cai, G.-R., Hu, X.-Y., Liu, J.O., 2006. Total synthesis of the cyclodepsipeptide apratoxin A and its analogues and assessment of their biological activities. Chemistry 12, 7615-7626.

[60] Marquez, B.L., Watts, K.S., Yokochi, A., Roberts, M.A., Verdier-Pinard, P., Jimenez, J.I., Hamel, E., Scheuer, P.J., Gerwick, W.H., 2002. Structure and absolute stereochemistry of hectochlorin, a potent stimulator of actin assembly. J. Nat. Prod. 65, 866-871.

[61] Gerwick WH, Proteau PJ, Nagle DG, Hamel E, Blokhin A & Slate DL (1994) Structure of curacin A, a novel

antimitotic, antiproliferative and brine shrimp toxic natural product from the marine cyanobacterium Lyngbya majuscula. J Org Chem 59: 1243-1245.

[62] Gerwick WH, Tan LT & Sitachitta N (2001) Nitrogen-containing metabolites from marine cyanobacteria. Alkaloids Chem Biol 57: 75-184.

[63] Glinski M, Hornbogen T & Zocher R (2001) Enzymatic synthesis of fungal N-methylated cyclopeptides and depsipeptides. Enzyme Technologies for Pharmaceutical and Biotechnological Applications (Kirts HA, Yeh W-K & Zmijewski MJ Jr, eds), Marcel Dekker, New York.

[64] Golakoti T, Ohtani I, Patterson DJ, Moore RE, Corbett TH, Valerlote FA & Demchik L (1994) Total structures of cryptophycins, potent antitumor depsipeptides from the blue- green alga Nostoc sp. strain GSV 224. J Am chem Soc 116: 4729-4737.

[65] Golakoti T, Ogino J, Heltzel CE, et al. (1995) Structure determination, conformational analysis, chemical stability studies, and antitumor evaluation of the cryptophycins. Isolation of 18 new analogs from Nostoc sp. strain GSV 224. J Am chem Soc 117: 12030-12049.

[66] Golakoti T, Yoshida WY, Chaganty S & Moore RE (2000) Isolation and structures of nostopeptolides A1, A2, and A3 from the cyanobacterium Nostoc sp. Tetrahedron 56: 9093-9102.

[67] Golakoti T, Yoshida WY, Chaganty S & Moore RE (2001) Isolation and structure determination of Nostocyclopeptides A1 and A2 from the terrestrial cyanobacterium Nostoc sp. ATCC53789. J Nat Prod 64: 54-59.

[68] Grach-Pogrebinsky O, Sedmak B & Carmeli S (2004) Seco[D- Asp3] microcystin-RR and [D-Asp3,D-Glu(OMe)6]microcystin-RR, two new microcystins from a toxic water bloom of the cyanobacterium Planktothrix rubescens. J Nat Prod 67: 337-342.

[69] Gregson JM, Chen J-L, Patterson GML & Moore RE (1992) Structures of puwainaphycins A-E. Tetrahedron 48: 3727-3734.

[70] Gross EM (1999) Allelopathy in benthic and littoral areas: case studies on allelochemicals from benthic cyanobacteria and submersed macrophytes. Principles and Practices in Plant Ecology (Dakshini KMM & Foy CF, eds), pp. 179-199. CRC Press, Boca Raton.

[71] Gross EM (2003) Allelopathy of aquatic autotrophs. Crit Rev Plant Sci 22: 313-339.

[72] Guenzi E, Galli G, Grgurina I, Gross DC & Grandi G (1998) Characterization of the syringomycin synthetase gene cluster. A link between prokaryotic and eukaryotic peptide synthetases. J Biol Chem 273: 32857-32863.

[73] Coleman, J.E.; van Soest, R.; Andersen, R.J. New geodiamolides from the sponge *Cymbastela* sp. collected in Papua New Guinea. *J. Nat. Prod.* **1999**, *62*, 1137-1141.

[74] Freitas, V.; Rangel, M.; Bisson, L.; Jaeger, R.; Machado-Santelli, G. The geodiamolide H, derived from Brazilian sponge *Geodia corticostylifera*, regulates actin cytoskeleton, migration and invasion of breast cancer cells cultured in three-dimensional environment. J. Cell. Physiol. **2008**, *216*, 583-594.

[75] Gamble, W.R.; Durso, N.A.; Fuller, R.W.; Westergaard, C.K.; Johnson, T.R.; Sackett, D.L.; Hamel, E.; Cardellina, J.H., II; Boyd, M.R. Cytotoxic and tubulin-interactive hemiasterlins from *Auletta* sp. and *Siphonochalina* spp. sponges. *Bioorg. Med.* Chem. **1999**, *7*, 1611-1615.

[76] Molinski, T.F.; Dalisay, D.S.; Lievens, S.L.; Saludes, J.P. Drug development from marine natural products. Nat. Rev. Drug. Discov. **2009**, *8*, 69-85.

[77] Talpir, R.; Benayahu, Y.; Kashman, Y.; Pannell, L.; Schleyer, M. Hemiasterlin and geodiamolide TA; two new cytotoxic peptides from the marine sponge *Hemiasterella minor* (Kirkpatrick). Tetrahedron Lett. **1994**, *35*, 4453-4456.

[78] Anderson, H.J.; Coleman, J.E.; Andersen, R.J.; Roberge, M. Cytotoxic peptides hemiasterlin, hemiasterlin A and hemiasterlin B induce mitotic arrest and abnormal spindle formation. Cancer Chemother. Pharmacol. **1997**, *39*, 223-226.

[79] Rocha-Lima, C.M.; Bayraktar, S.; Macintyre, J.; Raez, L.; Flores, A.M.; Ferrell, A.; Rubin, E.H.; Poplin, E.A.; Tan, A.R.; Lucarelli, A.; et al. A phase 1 trial of E7974 administered on day 1 of a 21-day cycle in patients with advanced solid tumors. Cancer **2012**, *118*, 4262-4270.

[80] Loganzo, F.; Discafani, C.M.; Annable, T.; Beyer, C.; Musto, S.; Hari, M.; Tan, X.; Hardy, C.; Hernandez, R.; Baxter, M.; et al. HTI-286, a synthetic analogue of the tripeptide hemiasterlin, is a potent antimicrotubule agent that circumvents p-glycoprotein-mediated resistance in vitro and in vivo. Cancer Res. **2003**, *63*, 1838-1845.

[81] Malloy, K.; Engene, N.; Pedler, B.; Clark, B.R.; Gerwick, W.H. Isolation, structure elucidation, and SAR perspectives of cyanobacterial cyclic depsipeptides containing the unique Dhoya (3- hydroxy-2,2-dimethyl-7-octynoic acid) fragment and its derivatives. In *42nd Western Regional Meeting of the American Chemical Society*, Las Vegas, NV, USA, September 2008.

[82] Kwan, J.C.; Rocca, J.R.; Abboud, K.A.; Paul, V.J.; Luesch, H. Total structure determination of grassypeptolide, a new marine cytotoxin. Org. Lett. **2008**, *10*, 789-792.

[83] Hawkins, C.J.; Lavin, M.F.; Marshall, K.A.; van den Brenk, A.L; Watters, D.J. Structure-activity relationships of the lissoclinamides: cytotoxic cyclic peptides from the ascidian *Lissoclinum patella*. J. Med. Chem. **1990**, *33*, 1634-1638.

[84] Wipf, P.; Fritch, P.C.; Geib, S.J.; Sefler, A.M. Conformational studies and structure–activity analysis of lissoclinamide 7 and related cyclopeptide alkaloids. J. Am. Chem. Soc. **1998**, *120*, 4105-4112.

[85] Gunasekera, S.P.; Ritson-Williams, R.; Paul, V.J. Carriebowmide, a new cyclodepsipeptide from the marine cyanobacterium *Lyngbya polychroa*. J. Nat. Prod. **2008**, *71*, 2060-2063.

[86] Silva ON, de la Fuente-Núñez C, Haney EF, et al. An anti-infective synthetic peptide with dual antimicrobial and immunomodulatory activities. Sci Rep. 2016;6:35465.

[87] Pereira, A.; Cao, Z.; Murray, T.F.; Gerwick, W.H. Hoiamide A, a sodium channel activator of unusual architecture from a consortium of two Pupa New guinea cyanobactiera. Chem. Biol. **2009**, *16*, 893-906.

Chapter 5

Molecular Pathogenesis of Inflammatory Cytokines in Insulin Resistance Diabetes Mellitus

Haamid Bashir, Mohammad Hayat Bhat and Sabhiya Majid

Abstract

Diabetes Mellitus Type 2 (T2DM) is a non-communicable and multifactorial disease. It is a leading cause of premature deaths worldwide. Inflammatory cytokines are reported that they have potential to enhance insulin resistance and hence T2DM. The current research was taken to investigate the possible role of inflammatory mediators: Tumor Necrosis Factor (TNF-α) and White blood cells (WBC's) in mobilizing biological molecules mainly immunological nature. A total of 320 subjects were selected in this study among them 160 were T2DM cases and 160 were healthy controls. Serum concentration of Tumor Necrosis Factor-a (TNF-α) was quantified by ELISA method, WBC count was measured on Sysmax (Germany) hematology analyzer, biochemical and Immunoassay parameters were done on fully automatic analyzers. The expression of candidate pro-inflammatory cytokine (TNF-α), and (WBC's) were elevated in T2DM. TNF-α shows association ($p<0.001$) with glycemic profile and insulin sensitivity in T2DM cases in comparison with healthy controls. Induction of inflammation and up regulation of pro-inflammatory cytokines has been purported to play a significant role in pathogenesis of T2DM and study confirms that the positive correlation of TNF-α with T2DM and hence to insulin sensitivity. These can act as early prediction biomarkers in diagnosis and prognosis of human disease i.e Diabetes Mellitus. Further studies are needed to help clinicians manage and treat T2DM effectively.

Keywords: inflammation, biomarkers, cytokines, mediators, type 2 diabetes mellitus

1. Introduction

The term Diabetes Mellitus describes a metabolic disorder of multiple etiologies characterized by chronic hyperglycemia accompanied by distressed metabolism of carbohydrates, fats and proteins resulting from defects in insulin secretion, insulin action or both [1]. Diabetes Mellitus (T2DM), is a non-communicable, chronic disorder and progresses slowly because of multifactorial etiology and is a leading cause of premature deaths worldwide, also, its exceptional upsurge poses a severe threat on human society and imposes a huge economic burden worldwide [2]. As per recent reports of World Health Organization (WHO), 422 million people globally are affected from the diabetes mellitus with a prevalence rate of 8.5% and 46.3% still remains undiagnosed and number is projected to rise 552 million in 2030

[3]. Furthermore, highly effected population are living in developing countries and comprises of 40–60 age group. In 2017, studies reported that India alone has 72 million people affected with T2DM and is projected to rise 101.2 million in 2030 [3, 4]. The risk factors of T2DM are suggestively increased with changing lifestyle, blood pressure, central obesity, inadequate physical activity and unhealthy diet [5] Blood glucose fasting (FBG), Two-hour post prandial blood glucose (Two-hour-PP) and glycated hemoglobin (HbA1c) levels are most widely used as glycemic control markers which indicates progression of the disease and development of its complications. Studies reported diabetes mellitus are T2DM linked with lipid and lipoprotein irregularities, including reduced HDL cholesterol and raised triglycerides [6–10].

Recent decade the diabetes mellitus, witnessed transformation from the epidemic to pandemic at global level. The global projections revealed that diabetes is affecting nearly 10% of the world's population [11]. As per reports of World Health Organization (WHO), the prevalence of diabetes mellitus is likely to increase by 35% by the year 2030-45 [11]. It is the most common form of the disease, accounting for about 90 to 95% of all diagnosed cases of diabetes. T2DM is a group of genetically determined diseases which may be controlled by diet and/or hypoglycemic agents and/or exogenous insulin [12]. Although, it is mainly characterized by insulin resistance, but impairment in insulin secretion also occurs later in type 2 diabetes mellitus [13]. It occurs usually in individuals over 30 years of age and dramatically increases as a result of changes in human behavior and increased body mass index [14]. The global rise in diabetes mellitus is referred to population growth, aging, increasing trends towards an unhealthy diet, obesity and modern lifestyles [15]. Inflammation can be classified as acute, high-grade, or chronic low-grade inflammation [16]. Acute inflammation is essential for survival, because it initiates pathogen killing, initiates tissue repair processes, and helps to restore homeostasis after infection or tissue damage [16]. In general, acute inflammatory responses are short-term responses [16]. When clinical manifestations are minimal or absent, it is classified as low-grade inflammation [16]. Low-grade inflammation is characterized by slightly elevated blood concentrations of acute-phase proteins, cytokines, and mediators with endothelial activation capacity that are involved in acute inflammation as well [16]. It is likely that dysfunction of adipose tissue is a major contributor to chronic low-grade inflammation [16]. Adipose tissue dysfunction, is characterized by a reduced capacity to store dietary lipids and an impaired endogenous lipolysis, leading to lipid overflow and ectopic fat accumulation, which has been related to the development of insulin resistance. Adipose tissue has a dual function, in addition to acting as a storage repository of the body system has role in endocrine function system, secretes the inflammatory markers. Thus, any sort of imbalance in the secretion leads to low grade inflammation. The matured adipocytes, as observed in individuals with overweight, relate among others to an higher secretion of the pro-inflammatory cytokines tumor necrosis factor-alpha (TNF-α) and interleukin-6 (IL-6) and a lower secretion of the anti-inflammatory cytokine, adipokine, adiponectin like IL-10. Besides secretion of cytokines by the adipocytes themselves, macrophages that infiltrate the obese adipose tissue can also secrete cytokines [17]. Being secreted, these pro-inflammatory cytokines can have autocrine and paracrine effects at the site of the adipose tissue [18]. Furthermore, these cytokines can be transported via the blood stream to act on distant targets, like the skeletal muscle and liver [18]. Besides adipose tissue, hyperglycemia itself can contribute to chronic-low grade inflammation. Hyperglycemia can stimulate the production of reactive oxygen species, which, in turn, stimulate production of pro-inflammatory cytokines, like TNF-α and IL-6 [19]. Insulin, however, could counterbalance the pro-inflammatory effect of glucose by suppressing the production of the pro-inflammatory cytokines and by activating the production of anti-inflammatory cytokines, like interleukin-4 and interleukin-10 [20]. Thus imbalance in cytokine expression can contribute to insulin resistance. TNF-α expression can affect the insulin signaling cascade by phosphorylation of the insulin receptor, insulin receptor substrate, and glucose transporter, can suppress expression of genes encoding for adiponectin, and can increase the expression of genes encoding for IL-6 [16, 20]. TNF-α and IL-6 also enhance oxidative stress by stimulation NF-kB or NADPH oxidase [19]. NF-kB causes a transcriptional response of genes involved in inflammatory processes. A high concentration of IL-6 stimulates the production of acute-phase protein C-reactive protein (CRP) in the liver [21]. CRP is a non-specific inflammation marker that may contribute to insulin resistance by increasing phosphorylation of IRS and by increasing the synthesis of cytokines like TNF-α and IL-6 [22]. In line with the proposed mechanisms, several prospective studies observed associations between slightly elevated concentrations of the inflammation markers CRP, TNF-α, and IL-6 and type 2 diabetes mellitus in different populations of world [23–25]. Weiyi et al. reported that circulating antibodies in plasma against inflammatory cytokines are associated with type 2 diabetes mellitus. Furthermore, some prospective cohort studies showed that participants with higher CRP, TNF-α, or IL-6 concentration had a higher risk of type 2 diabetes [26, 27].

Inclination of T2DM from metabolic disorder to inflammation is changed due to variations in pro and anti- inflammatory cytokines like tumor necrosis factor alpha-α (TNF-α), interleukin-6 (IL-6) and C-reactive protein (CRP) [26]. It has been reported in insulin signaling pathways, cross linking and ultimately developing insulin resistance in β-cells of pancreas which further risks to T2DM [28, 29]. Steadiness among these pro and anti-inflammatory cytokines is compulsory to make β-cells immune to any infection which may lead to T2DM [30].

This chapter will focus on the studies about the role of, proinflammatory cytokine in diabetes mellitus.

2. Role of inflammatory mediators in T2DM

Numerous studies demonstrated that, the various inflammatory mediators in type 2 diabetes mellitus (T2DM), has been found abnormally high levels of cytokines, plasminogen activator inhibitor, chemokines, acute phase proteins (such as CRP) [24, 31]. The elevated concentrations of pro-inflammatory cytokines (TNF-α, IL-6 and CRP) initiates the activation of innate immune system in type 2 diabetic patients due to over-nutrition. Nutrients comprises of elements necessary for body functioning and development are minerals, vitamins, fats, carbohydrates, and proteins. Inflammatory mediators and CRPs, are considered to vary from individual to individual and tissue to tissue. In patients with T2DM, increased circulating levels of various proinflammatory cytokines and chemokines have been detected [32]. Consequently, one may not predict the degree and extent of inflammation in specific tissue by only observing the circulating levels of these pro-inflammatory mediators, which eradicates β-cells themselves leading to β-cell dysfunction.

2.1 Cytokines

The cytokines coined from two Greek words, "*cyto*" means cavity or cell" and "*kines*" means movement. They are soluble proteins with low molecular weight proteins <30 kD, secreted by the cells of the bothinnate and adaptive immunity. These cytokines are chemically peptide molecules, and cannot cross the lipid bilayer of cells to enter the cytoplasm. Cytokines have high affinity for receptors and are active in 'picomole' concentration. They function as autocrine, paracrine and endocrine signaling. Based on cellular sources there are three types of cytokines:- Monokines (*mononuclear phagocyte*), lymphokines (*lymphocytes*), interleukins (*leukocytes*) (TNF, IL-6, IL-10 etc.). In addition, a subfamily of cytokines called chemokines, which functions in directing migration of cells. Cytokines are produced by a wide series of immune cells, like macrophages, B lymphocytes, T lymphocytes and mast cells. They act through receptors, in the immune system. Cytokines modulate the balance between humoral and cell-based immune responses, and they regulate the maturation, growth, and responsiveness of particular cell populations. Cytokines has been classed as lymphokines, interleukins, and chemokines, based on, cell of secretion, or target of action. Because cytokines have important characteristics of redundancy and pleiotropism. Cytokines are the key modulators of inflammation, participating in acute and chronic inflammation.

2.2 Tumor necrosis factor (TNF-α)

The term tumor-necrosis factor, which is abbreviated as TNF. TNF, is primarily produced as a 233-amino acid long type II transmembrane protein arranged in stable homotrimers. The TNF-α gene is present as a single copy gene on human chromosome 6 located on position (6p21.33). The gene consists of four exons and three introns. Interestingly, more than 80% of the mature TNF-α sequence is encoded in the fourth exon. Tumor necrosis factor (TNF-α) was initially identified in the 1970s as an endotoxin-induced serum factor responsible for the necrosis of certain tumours *in vivo* and *in vitro*. Subsequently, TNF-α was isolated and its gene was cloned. TNF-α, is an essential signaling protein in the innate and adaptive immune systems. It plays important role in tissue degeneration and repair. It stimulates the proliferation of normal cells, exerts cytolytic or cytostatic activity against tumor cells, and causes inflammatory, antiviral, and immunoregulatory effects.

TNF-α also performs in additional functions linked with lipid metabolism, coagulation, insulin resistance, and endothelial function. TNF-α is the prototypic member of the TNF superfamily of type II trans-membrane proteins that includes 30 receptors and 19 associated ligands with diverse functions in cell differentiation, inflammation, immunity and apoptosis. It is primarily secreted from activated macrophages, although it may also be secreted by other cell types including monocytes, T-cells, mast cells, NK-cells, keratinocytes, fibroblasts and neurons (Tracey et al., 2008). TNF-α is synthesized as a transmembrane precursor protein (m-TNF-α) with a molecular mass of 26 kDa, it is transported *via* the rough endoplasmic reticulum (RER), Golgi complex and the recycling endosome to the cell surface. The monomers of TNF-α associate at the plasma membrane as non-covalent trimmers prior to being cleaved by the metalloprotease, TNF-α converting enzyme(TACEorADAM17) (Black et al., 1997). Cleavage by TACE results in the production of 17 kDa soluble TNF-α (sTNFα) ectodomain and it is trimers of sTNFα that constitute the potent ligand that activates TNF receptors. Following TACE cleavage, the membrane proteolytically processed by the signal peptide peptidases (SPPLs) SPPL2a and SPPL2b. This cleavage produces an intra cellular domain (ICD) that translocates to the nucleus and induces pro-inflammatory cytokine signaling. Thus, the precursor TNF-α molecule is subjected to multiple cleavage events to release potent modulators of inflammation. TNF-α, is a pleiotropic cytokine which signals through two receptors: TNF receptor 1 (TNFR1) and TNF receptor 2 (TNFR2). The receptors are expressed on different cell types, with TNFR1 being widely expressed, while TNFR2 is expressed predominantly on leukocytes and endothelial cells. The two TNFRs have been reported to mediate distinct biological effects. Both TNFR1 and TNFR2 are single transmembrane glycoproteins with 28% homology in their extracellular domains (**Figure 1**).

It comprises of four cysteine-rich domains (CRDs), each of which comprises three cysteine-cysteine disulphide bonds, and a pre- ligand binding assembly domain (PLAD) involved in trimerisation of the receptor. Importantly, the receptors differ by the presence of an intracellular death domain (DD) at the carboxyl-end of TNFR1, that is able to drive either apoptosis or inflammation through interaction with associated adaptor molecules (**Figure 1**). Recruitment of TRADD to TNFR1 is required for both signaling pathways. Subsequently, one of two complexes is formed, either at the cell surface (complex-I) or following internalization (complex-II). The formation of complex-I requires TNFR-associated factor 2 (TRAF2) and receptor- interacting protein (RIP), leading to kinase cascades that trigger pro- inflammatory gene expression. Alternatively, should the first complex fail to signal, Complex II is formed to induce apoptosis. In Complex II, proteolysis and internalization of the receptor results in the recruitment of FADD and pro-caspase-8 to form the death-inducing signaling complex. The distinct cytoplasmic domains could account for the differential signaling of the receptors by sTNFα and mTNFα. It was found that mTNFα was a more potent activator of TNFR2 than sTNFα and induced distinct biological outcomes. Further, activation of TNFR1 was found to

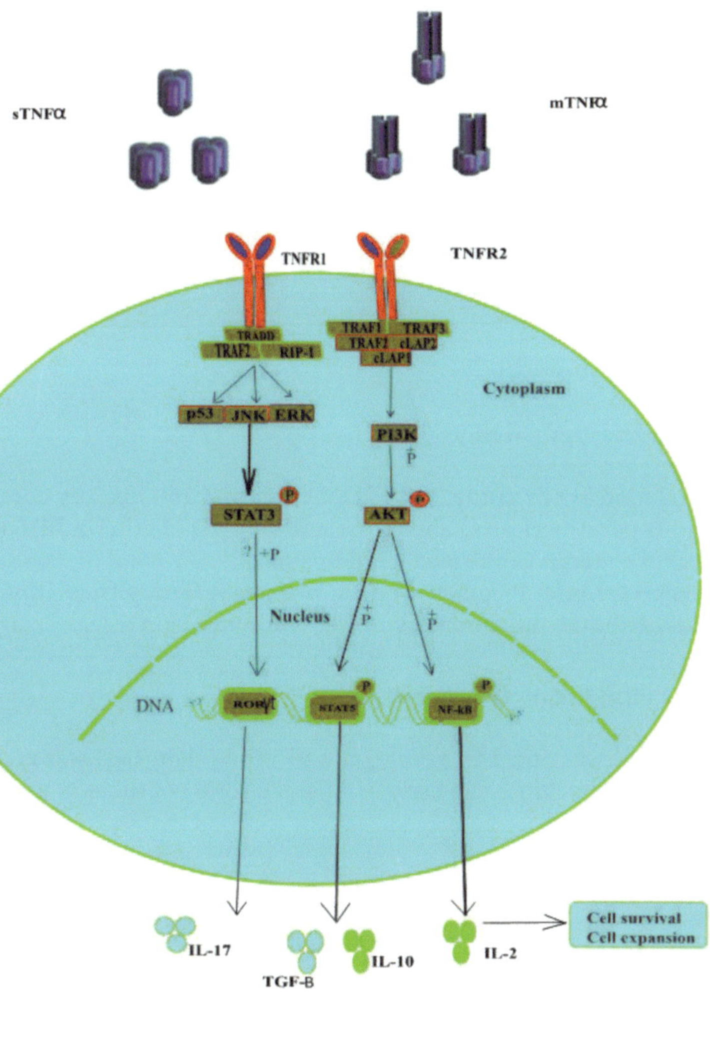

Figure 1.
Mechanism of TNF-α receptors and association with other inflammatory cytokines (source: Sujuan et al., 2018. Front. Immunol; 9:784).

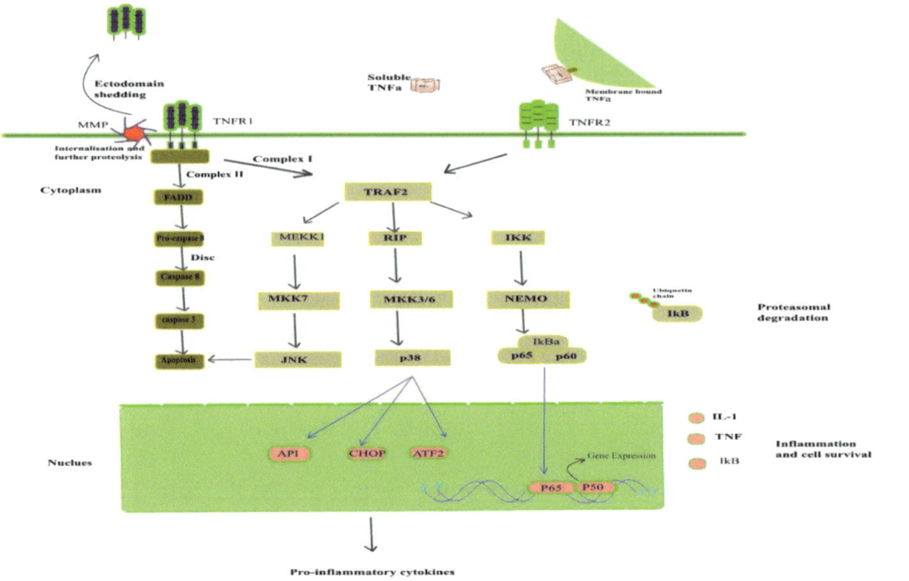

Figure 2.
Mechanism of TNF receptor1 and 2, activating signaling pathways of pro-inflammatory cytokines (source: Ana Falvia et al., 2019. World J Gastrointest Oncol. Apr 15, 2019; 11(4): 281–294).

stimulate NF-κB expression to a significantly greater extent than TNFR2. Finally, Scatchard analysis of ligand binding to TNFR1 and TNFR2 found that the former had a higher affinity for TNF-α. Thus, TNFR1 is considered to be the more important of the two receptors for the activation of pro- inflammatory signaling pathways (**Figure 2**).

3. Materials and methods

3.1 Subjects and study design

We included in our study 340 T2DM cases and 160 healthy controls, 30–60-years old as per American Diabetes Association (ADA) criteria 2016 (**Table 1**).

Inclusion criteria: Confirmed T2DM patients.

Exclusion criteria: Pregnant women, patients suffering from (thyroiditis, rheumatoid arthritis, inflammatory bowel syndrome, skin diseases, any cancer).

3.2 Anthropometric measurement

Height (cm) was noted by a scale on wall and Weight (kg) was measured by digital weighing machine. The body mass index (BMI) of subjects was calculated by

FBG ≥126 mg/dl. Fasting means no food ingestion for ≥ 8 hours
2-hr BG ≥200 mg/dl
HbA1C ≥6.5%.
Random BG ≥200 mg/dl.

Table 1.
American Diabetes Association (ADA) 2016 criteria for diagnosing T2DM.

formulae = weight (Kg) / height (m^2). Participants with a BMI ≥30.0 kg/m^2 were considered obese as per NCEP ATPIII criteria. "Waist circumference" (WC) was evaluated in the middle, between the lower rib margin and the iliac crest with subjects in upright position.

3.3 Biochemical and immunoassay analysis

Glycated hemoglobin (HbA1c) levels and clinical chemistry was evaluated for all cases and healthy controls. The Insulin resistance (IR) of subjects was accepted by calculating the index of HOMA-IR (homeostatic model assessment – insulin resistance) which is as under: "**HOMA-IR = fasting insulin (µU/ml) × fasting glucose (mg/dl)/405**" (24). Following HOMA-IR score was used as reference range for classification of IR.

- < 3 = Normal IR b) Between 3 and 5 = Moderate IR c) >5 = Severe IR

White Blood Cell count analysis: whole Blood samples were taken in EDTA vials were analyzed for WBC count on Sysmax hematology analyzer (Germany).

Estimation of Pro-inflammatory cytokine (TNF-α) by Enzyme linked Immunoassay (ELISA) Analysis.

TNF-α assay: Quantitative measurement of TNF- α was done by 'Diaclone Human TNF-α ELISA kit' (France).

Statistical analysis: Data was compiled on Microsoft excel 2011 spread sheet. All the data were expressed as a mean ± standard deviation and significance value (p) were calculated. Data analysis were performed by using statistical 'software SPSS 16.1' (Chicago, IL). Students T-test was done on biochemical, immunoassay and inflammatory mediators. Chi-square test was done on socio-demographic characters. Correlation analysis was performed for determining the association between serum TNF-α, and other parameters, Pearson correlation coefficient (r) was obtained. $P < 0.05$ were considered statistically significant.

4. Result and discussion

Total 320 subjects were included for the study among 160 were cases and 160 were controls (**Table 2**). The mean ± SD age of cases were (49.9 ± 9.4) Years and that of healthy controls were (46.9 ± 9.9) years which is statistically significant (p = 0.003). In this study, It was observed that BMI was (42.2 ± 8.1) kg/m^2 in T2DM cases and in healthy controls was (21.2 ± 2.2) kg/m^2 which is statistically significant (p = 0.003). Among 160 cases 81 were males and 79 females and in healthy controls 80 were males and 80 were females, on gender wise comparison difference in patients and controls are significant (p = 0.005).

In **Table 3**, biochemical profile of T2DM cases and healthy controls were summarized and it was found that there were increase trend in parameters of lipid

Variables	T2DM Cases (n = 160)	Controls (n = 160)	p value
Age (Years)	49.9 ± 9.4	46.9 ± 9.9	0.003
Gender (M/F)	81/79	80/80	0.005
BMI (kg/m^2)	42.2 ± 8.1	21.2 ± 2.2	0.002

Table 2.
Anthropometric analysis in study subjects.

Variables	Diabetes mellitus (n = 160)	Controls (n = 160)	p value
Fasting Glucose (mg/dl)	168.4 ± 32.7	81.9 ± 7.7	0.119
Post-parandial Glucose (mg/dl)	316.2 ± 51.6	122.1 ± 9.1	0.001
Total Cholesterol (mg/dl)	298.5 ± 54.1	109.1 ± 27.9	0.002
Triglycerides (mg/dl)	319.5 ± 57.1	146.1 ± 29.6	0.003
HDL (mg/dl)	92.4 ± 22.6	52.9 ± 10.1	0.024
LDL (mg/dl)	148.3 ± 9.1	69.8 ± 29.8	0.002
HBA1c (%)	9.9 ± 2.8	4.9 ± 0.8	0.014

Table 3.
Levels of clinical chemistry parameters in study group.

profile like serum Triglycerides (TG), total cholesterol (TC), Low Density Lipoprotein (LDL) and High Density Lipoprotein (HDL) among T2DM cases as compared to healthy controls and the trend were significantly high ($p < 0.05$). The glycemic profile (Glucose Fasting and HbA1c) in T2DM cases was higher as compared to healthy controls and are found to be statistically significant ($p < 0.05$).

Figure 3, Histogram representing graphical analysis of Insulin and HOMA-IR of study group where there was elevation in the Insulin (μU/ml) levels among T2DM case (32.6 ± 7.5) as compared to healthy controls (7.8 ± 2.1) and it was found that the elevation level among the T2DM cases was significantly ($p = 0.001$) higher than healthy controls. The HOMA-IR index for insulin sensitivity was calculated by a standard formula in both T2DM cases and healthy controls and was found significantly ($p < 0.05$) higher in T2DM cases. **Table 4**, describes the levels of serum inflammatory mediators (TNF-α, and WBC) in T2DM cases and healthy controls; the mean ± SD value of inflammatory markers in T2DM cases was as WBC = 8495 ± 1943, TNF-α = 36.5 ± 7.8 while in healthy controls it was WBC =7389 ± 1504, TNF-α =13.7 ± 4.4 and it was found that in T2DM patients the levels of inflammatory mediators were highly significant ($p < 0.05$) in comparison with healthy controls.

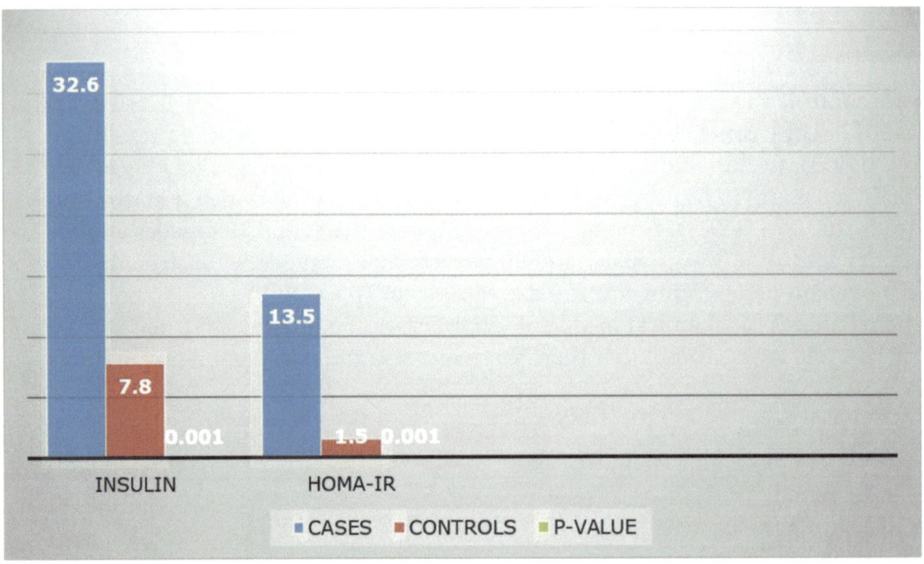

Figure 3.
Histogram representing immunoassay analysis of study group.

Variables	Diabetes mellitus (n = 160)	Controls (n = 160)	p value (<0.05)
TLC (thousands)	8495 ± 1943	7389 ± 1504	0.002
TNF-α (pg/ml)	36.5 ± 7.8	13.7 ± 4.4	0.002

Table 4.
Levels of inflammatory mediators in the study group.

Inflammatory mediators	Male T2DM (n = 81)	Female T2DM (n = 79)	Male controls (n = 80)	Female controls (n = 80)	p-value <0.05
TNF-α (pg/dl)	8.8 ± 0.8	8.7 ± 1.0	3.6 ± 0.5	3.7 ± 0.4	0.001
WBC (thousands)	1974 ± 206	1784 ± 184	1459 ± 169	1385 ± 165	0.082

Table 5.
Comparison of inflammatory mediators in T2DM male and female patients versus control subjects.

Table 5 shows the comparison of inflammatory mediators within gender groups and it was found that in female cases levels of inflammatory mediators was highly significant ($p < 0.05$) as compared to male cases while WBC was not statistically significant, which provides us the information that females may be at higher risk to T2DM.

Figures 4–7 shows the correlation of inflammatory mediators in T2DM cases and controls with glycemic profile and insulin sensitivity and was studied by Pearson's correlation analysis. TNF- α shows positive correlation with glycemic profile (Glucose fasting, HbA1c) and insulin sensitivity (Insulin assay, HOMA-IR) in T2DM cases and were statistically significant ($p < 0.05$).

Table 6, describes the relationship of inflammatory mediators with glycemic profile and the **Table 7**, depicts the relationship of insulin sensitivity as per gender wise in cases and controls. We observed in Males and Female T2DM cases there was a positive correlation ($p = 0.001$) of TNF-α with glycemic profile and Insulin sensitivity and other inflammatory mediators show negative and weak correlation. Worldwide people are suffering from T2DM and it is projected to increase from

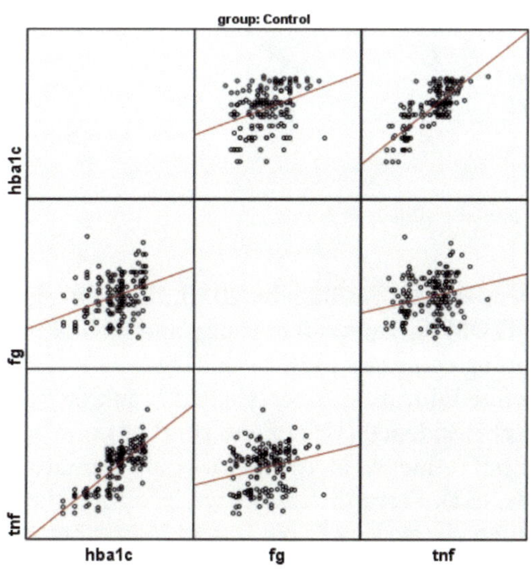

Figure 4.
Correlation of TNF-α with glycemic profile in controls.

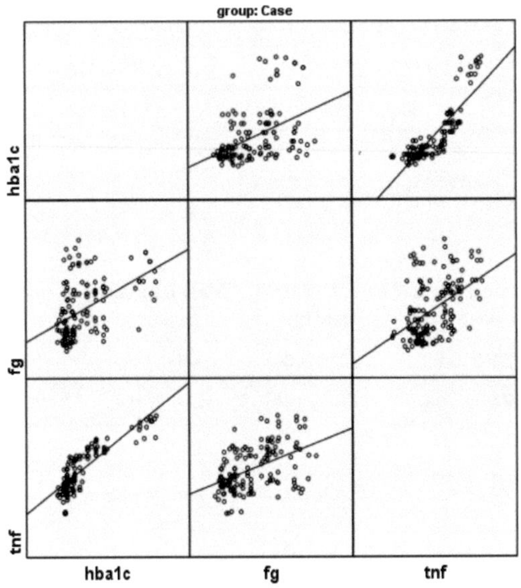

Figure 5.
Correlation of TNF-α with glycemic profile in cases.

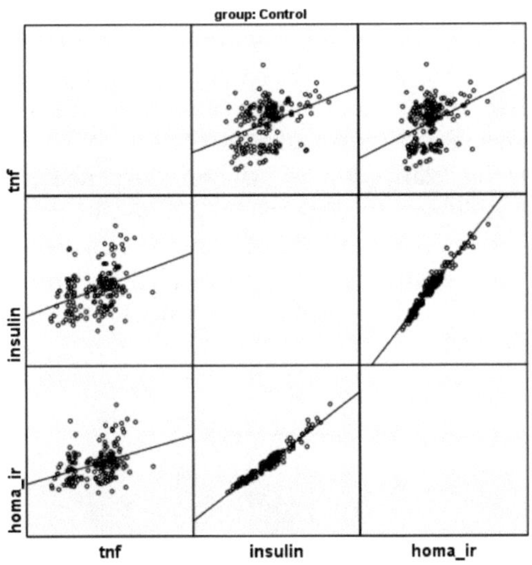

Figure 6.
Correlation of TNF-α with insulin sensitivity in controls.

present 415 million people to 642 million by 2040. In all developing countries it was seen that number of T2DM patients is increasing and 75% of people with T2DM are living in these developing countries [33]. In this study, we observed that Socio-Demographic factors like Education, Lifestyle and Smoking has significant association with T2DM except Residence (Urban and rural of same geographical area) which had no substantial influence on the levels of inflammatory mediators of study like, TNF-α, and WBC (32). From the results we infer that there were increased expression of inflammatory markers (TNF-α, and WBC) between cases and controls which supports the findings of Phosat, et al. [34] as they found in their study that there were greater risk of T2DM with higher levels of inflammatory mediators [34]. On comparison between sex wise within case group it was

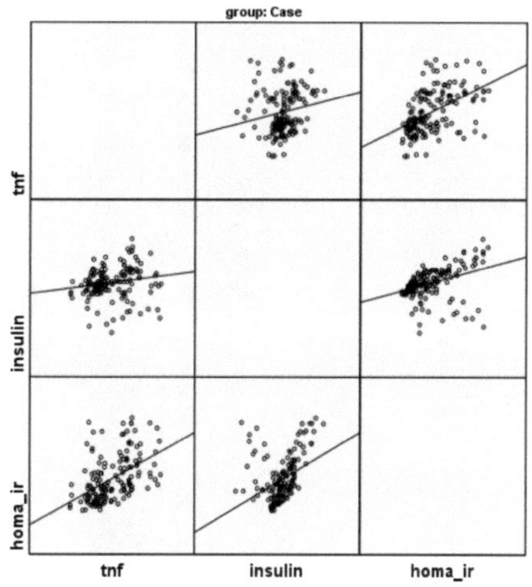

Figure 7.
Correlation of TNF-α with insulin sensitivity in cases.

observed that there was an elevation in levels of TNF-α in Female T2DM cases as compared to Male T2DM Cases which are in agreement with the findings of Insha et al., [9, 10, 33, 35]. There are many research studies on this subject which demonstrated that levels of markers of inflammatory reactions increased with the decrease in insulin sensitivity depending on the severity of T2DM [36, 37]. In this study both Male and Female sexes have confirmed the importance of inflammatory mediators in the pathogenesis of T2DM. The levels of TNF-α rise significantly in both sexes compared to control group showing correlation with glycemic profile and Insulin sensitivity thus, being considered an independent predictor of risk of developing T2DM [34].

This study experimentally determined that only pro-inflammatory cytokine TNF-α can leads to pathogenesis of T2DM while other inflammatory cytokines shows negative and weak correlation with T2DM. This research study showed vibrant changes in concentrations of pro-inflammatory cytokines, in T2DM. Our findings are in concurrence with the results of [32], which showed serum expression of candidate mediators (TNF-α) are elevated in T2DM cases which are independent of physical activity and other risk factors [38]. It is suggest that TNF-α is an important predictor for the development of T2DM for Male and female, in both rural and urban populations.

Interestingly, results of our study showed a high degree of correlation between these promising cytokines (TNF, WBC) in T2DM in comparison to healthy controls. The results are statically significant. In this case–control study, we found in our T2DM cases there were significantly higher concentration of TNF-α as compared to those of controls which may be the possible cause of low grade inflammation and predisposes subjects to the T2DM or towards its complications. These assertions aggress with the findings of AL-Shukaili, et al. [39]. Furthermore our experimental finding provides evidence that the pattern and variation of these cytokines (TNF-α, and WBC) are important in the pathogenesis of T2DM [32]. Significant correlation of TNF-α inflammatory mediator in T2DM cases with glycemic profile and insulin sensitivity leads to pathogenesis of diseases in this ethnic population [32]. These findings are in agreement with the fact that inflammatory reactions depends on group of cytokines rather than a single one. The reports of inflammation has a role in pathogenesis of T2DM has been elucidated in several studies in different populations.

Inflammatory mediators	Cases				Controls			
	HBA1c		Fasting glucose		HBA1c		Fasting glucose	
	Males n = 81	Females n = 79	Males n = 81	Females n = 79	Males n = 80	Females n = 80	Males n = 80	Females n = 80
TNF-α	*p = 0.02 *r = 0.89	p = 0.003 r = 0.883	p = 0.004 r = 0.459	p = 0.005 r = 0.546	*p = 0.035 *r = 0.388	p = 0.011 r = 0.368	p = 0.013 r = 0.260	p = 0.063 r = 0.211

Table 6.
Pearson correlation coefficients of inflammatory mediators with glycemic profile, sex-wise.

Inflammatory mediators	Insulin		HOMA-IR		Insulin		HOMA-IR	
	Males n = 81	Females n = 79	Males n = 81	Females n = 79	Males n = 80	Females n = 80	Males n = 80	Females n = 80
TNF-α	*p = 0.008 *r = 0.478	p = 0.009 r = 0.368	p = 0.008 r = 0.374	p = 0.004 r = 0.388	*p = 0.012 *r = 0.016	p = 0.011 r = 0.019	p = 0.111 r = 0.099	p = 0.008 r = 0.319

Table 7.
Pearson correlation coefficients of inflammatory mediators with insulin sensitivity (sex-wise).

5. Conclusion

The study findings confirms that TNF-α, plays a positive role in the pathogenesis of T2DM and can act as early prediction biomarkers which can prevent T2DM in this population. Further studies on the wider range of inflammatory mediators in association with other biochemical, immunoassay and hematological parameters are needed to establish role of inflammatory markers as early prediction biomarkers which can prevent T2DM.

6. Highlights of chapter

1. Inflammation is initiated by trauma or injury, infection, and hence effects cascades of numerous cytokines and white blood cells. The low grade inflammation triggers inflammatory cells like neutrophils, macrophages and monocytes in blood stream and also expresses the pro-inflammatory cytokines like Tumor necrosis factor-alpha, and interleukin-6.

2. The liver cells synthesize acute-phase proteins under the stimulus of some cytokines, which flow through the bloodstream, reach the site of inflammation, and eradicate the pathogens through opsonization and eliciting the complement pathways.

3. The variations in the serum concentrations of TNF-α leads to pathogenesis of T2DM.

4. Diagnostic routine tests are sometimes invasive. To augment the modern diagnostics in patient care, the employment of noninvasive biomarkers are needed.

5. Molecular biological tools have modernized the field of the biomarkers. For the development of biomarkers, genomics and proteomics, pathophysiology of a disease are needed to understand, the most available technique is correlating serologic markers with clinical parameters.

Author details

Haamid Bashir[1*], Mohammad Hayat Bhat[2] and Sabhiya Majid[1]

1 Department of Biochemistry, Government Medical College Srinagar-Research Centre University of Kashmir, India

2 Department of Endocrinology Super-Specialty Hospital, Government Medical College Srinagar, India

*Address all correspondence to: haamidb7@gmail.com

References

[1] WHO. Definition and Diagnosis of Diabetes Mellitus and Intermediate Hyperglycaemia: Report of a WHO/IDF Consultation. 2006. Available from: https://apps.who.int/iris/handle/10665/43588

[2] Rashid T, Bhat S, Wani MU, et al. The lipid peroxidation and antioxidant status of type 2 diabetic patients in Kashmir (India). International Journal of Diabetes in Developing Countries. 2015;**35**:476–481. DOI: 10.1007/s13410-015-0320-5

[3] World Health Organization. Global Health Estimates: Deaths by Cause, Age, Sex and Country, 2000–2012. Geneva: WHO; 2014. Pubmed

[4] Farooq R, Majid S, Bhat SA, Amin S, Bhat MH, Wani HA, et al. Association of adiponectin gene polymorphism with type 2 diabetes and metabolic syndrome. Translational Metabolic Syndrome Research. 2018;**1**:39e47. Pubmed

[5] Waqas S, Tahir A, Nadeem SB, Mohammad R, Abdul H. Effect of diet on type 2 diabetes mellitus: A review. International Journal of Health Sciences. 2017;**11**(2):22. Pubmed

[6] Bhat MA, Bhat SA, Ahmad SB, Qureshi W, Majid S, Ali A. Biochemical profile and genetic polymorphism of MTHFRC677T in risk of type 2 diabetes mellituss. International Journal of Diabetes and Endocrinology. 2017;**2**(2):19-25. Pubmed

[7] Ali A, Ayaz A, Dar MA, Singh N, Bhat SA. A key role of insulin in diabetes mellitus. International Journal of Scientific Research in Science, Engineering and Technology. 2017;**3**(6):80-85. Medline

[8] Singh PS, Sharma H, Zafar KS, Singh PK, Yadav SK, Gautam RK. Prevalence of type 2 diabetes mellitus in rural population of India- a study from Western Uttar Pradesh. International Journal of Research in Medical Sciences. 2017;**5**(4):1363-1367. Pubmed

[9] Bashir H, Ahmad Bhat S, Majid S, Hamid R, Koul RK, Rehman MU, et al. Role of inflammatory mediators (TNF-α, IL-6, CRP), biochemical and hematological parameters in type 2 diabetes mellitus patients of Kashmir, India. Medical Journal of the Islamic Republic of Iran. 2020a;**12**(34):5. DOI: 10.34171/mjiri.34.5. PMID: 32284929; PMCID: PMC7139256

[10] Bashir H, Ahmad Bhat S, Majid S, Hamid R, Koul RK, Rehman MU, et al. Role of inflammatory mediators (TNF-α, IL-6, CRP), biochemical and hematological parameters in type 2 diabetes mellitus patients of Kashmir, India. Medical Journal of the Islamic Republic of Iran. 2020b;**12**(34):5. DOI: 10.34171/mjiri.34.5

[11] Saeedi P, Petersohn I, Salpea P, Malanda B, Karuranga S, Unwin N, et al. Global and regional diabetes prevalence estimates for 2019 and projections for 2030 and 2045: Results from the International Diabetes Federation Diabetes Atlas, 9th edition. Diabetes Research and Clinical Practice. 2019;**157**:107843. DOI: 10.1016/j.diabres.2019.107843. Epub 2019 Sep 10

[12] Groop LC. The molecular genetics of non-insulin-dependent diabetes mellitus. Journal of Internal Medicine. 1997;**241**(2):95-101

[13] Lebovitz HE. Insulin resistance: Definition and consequences. Experimental and Clinical Endocrinology & Diabetes. 2001;**109** (Suppl 2):S135-S148

[14] Elmer L. Cognitive issues in Parkinson's disease. Neurologic Clinics. 2004;**22**(3 Suppl):S91-S106

[15] Ahmed MF, Kazim SM, Ghori SS, et al. Antidiabetic activity of vinca rosea extracts in Alloxan-induced diabetic rats. International Journal of Endocrinology. 2010;**2010**:841090. DOI: 10.1155/2010/841090

[16] Calder PC. Feeding the immune system. Proceedings of the Nutrition Society. 2013;**72**(3):299-309

[17] Harford KA, Reynolds CM, McGillicuddy FC, Roche HM. Fats, inflammation and insulin resistance: Insights to the role of macrophage and T-cell accumulation in adipose tissue. Proceedings of the Nutrition Society. 2011;**70**(4):408-417

[18] Karastergiou K, Mohamed-Ali V. The autocrine and paracrine roles of adipokines. Molecular and Cellular Endocrinology. 2010;**318**(1-2):69-78

[19] Das M, Pal S, Ghosh A. Family history of type 2 diabetes and prevalence of metabolic syndrome in adult Asian Indians. Journal of Cardiovascular Disease Research. 2012; **3**(2):104-108

[20] Calle MC, Fernandez ML. Inflammation and type 2 diabetes. Diabetes & Metabolism. 2012;**38**(3): 183-191

[21] Pepys MB, Hirschfield GM. C-reactive protein: A critical update. Journal of Clinical Investigation. 2003; **111**(12):1805-1812. DOI: 10.1172/JCI18921. Erratum in: J Clin Invest. 2003 Jul;112(2):299

[22] Bello G, Cailotto F, Hanriot D, Kolopp-Sarda MN, Latger-Cannard V, Hess K, et al. C-reactive protein (CRP) increases VEGF-A expression in monocytic cells via a PI3-kinase and ERK 1/2 signaling dependent pathway. Atherosclerosis. 2008;**200**(2):286-293

[23] Schmidt MI, Duncan BB, Vigo A, Pankow JS, Couper D, Ballantyne CM, et al. Leptin and incident type 2 diabetes: risk or protection? Diabetologia. 2006;**49**(9):2086-2096

[24] Herder C, Illig T, Rathmann W, Martin S, Haastert B, Müller-Scholze S, et al. Inflammation and type 2 diabetes: Results from KORA Augsburg. Gesundheitswesen. 2005;**67**(Suppl 1): S115-S121

[25] Kolb H, Mandrup-Poulsen T. An immune origin of type 2 diabetes? Diabetologia. 2005;**48**(6):1038-1050. DOI: 10.1007/s00125-005-1764-9. Epub 2005 Apr 30. Erratum in: Diabetologia. 2005 Aug;48(8):1677

[26] Iqra H, Shariq RM, Shahnaz AM, Mudasar N, Khalid G, Bashir AG. Type 2 diabetes mellitus: From a metabolic disorder to an inflammatory condition. World Journal of Diabetes. 2015;**6**(4): 598-612. Pubmed

[27] Dehghan A, van Hoek M, Sijbrands EJ, Stijnen T, Hofman A, Witteman JC. Risk of type 2 diabetes attributable to C-reactive protein and other risk factors. Diabetes Care. 2007;**30**(10):2695-2699

[28] Arora P, Garcia-Bailo B, Dastani Z, Brenner D, Villegas A, Malik S, et al. Genetic polymorphisms of innate immunity-related inflammatory pathways and their association with factors related to type 2 diabetes. BMC Medical Genetics. 2011;**12**:95. Pubmed

[29] Belfki H, Ben Ali S, Bougatef S, Ben Ahmed D, Haddad N, Jmal A, et al. Association between C-reactive protein and type 2 diabetes in a Tunisian population. Inflammation. 2012;**35**: 684-689. Pubmed

[30] Dongway AC, Faggad AS, Zaki HY, Abdalla BE. C-reactive protein is associated with low-density lipoprotein cholesterol and obesity in type 2 diabetic Sudanese. Diabetes, Metabolic Syndrome and Obesity: Targets and Therapy. 2015;**8**:427-435. Pubmed

[31] Pradhan AD, Manson JE, Rifai N, Buring JE, Ridker PM. C-reactive protein, interleukin 6, and risk of developing type 2 diabetes mellitus. JAMA. 2001;**286**:327-334. Pubmed

[32] Akash MSH, Rehman K, Liaqat A. Tumor necrosis factor-alpha: Role in development of insulin resistance and pathogenesis of type 2 diabetes mellitus. Journal of Cellular Biochemistry. 2018; **119**(1):105-110

[33] Biradar SB, Desai AS, Kashinakunti SV, Rangappa M, Kallaganada GS, Devaranavadagi B. Correlation between glycemic control markers and lipid profile in type 2 diabetes mellitus and impaired glucose tolerance. International Journal of Advances in Medicine. 2018;**5**(4):832-837. Pubmed

[34] Phosat C, Panprathip P, Chumpathat N, et al. Elevated C-reactive protein, interleukin 6, tumor necrosis factor alpha and glycemic load associated with type 2 diabetes mellitus in rural Thais: A cross-sectional study. BMC Endocrine Disorders. 2017;**17**(1): 44. Pubmed

[35] Inshah D, Sabhiya M, Fouzia R, et al. Combinatorial effect of leptin, tumor necrosis factor-αlpha, and vitamin D in progression of type 2 diabetes in Kashmiri population. Asian Journal of Pharmaceutical and Clinical Research. 2018;**10**(11):477-482. Medline

[36] Lukic L, Lalic NM, Rajkovic N, Jotic A, Lalic K, Milicic T, et al. Hypertension in obese type 2 diabetes patients is associated with increases in insulin resistance and IL-6 cytokine levels: Potential targets for an efficient preventive intervention. International Journal of Environmental Research and Public Health. 2014a;**11**(4):3586-3598. Pubmed

[37] Lukic L, Lalic NM, Rajkovic N, Jotic A, Lalic K, Milicic T, et al. Hypertension in obese type 2 diabetes patients is associated with increases in insulin resistance and IL-6 cytokine levels: Potential targets for an efficient preventive intervention. International Journal of Environmental Research and Public Health. 2014b;**11**(4):3586-3598. Pubmed

[38] Samuel ND, Denis DY, Ellis OD, et al. Variations in levels of IL-6 and TNF-α in type 2 diabetes mellitus between rural and urban Ashanti Region of Ghana. BMC Endocrine Disorders. 2015;**15**(50):1-7. Pubmed

[39] Al-Shukaili A, Al-Ghafri S, Al-Marhoobi S, Al-Abri S, Al-Lawati J, Al-Maskari M. Analysis of inflammatory mediators in type 2 diabetes patients. International Journal of Endocrinology. 2013;**2013**:976810. DOI: 10.1155/2013/976810. Epub 2013 May 20. PM. ID: 23762057; PMCID: PMC3671680

Chapter 6

Mass Spectrometry (Imaging) for Detection and Identification of Cyclic AMPs: Focus on Human Neutrophil Peptides (HNPs)

Eline Berghmans and Geert Baggerman

Abstract

Antimicrobial peptides (AMPs) are known best for their role in innate immunity against bacteria, viruses, parasites and fungi. However, not only are they showing increasing promise as potential antimicrobial drug candidates, recently, it has been reported that certain AMPs also show a cytotoxic effect against cancer cells. Their possible antitumor effect could make AMPs interesting candidate cancer biomarkers and a possible lead for new anticancer therapy. Due to their cyclic structure, detection and identification of AMPs is challenging, however, mass spectrometry (imaging; MSI) has been shown as a powerful tool for visualization and identification of (unknown) cyclic AMPs. In this chapter, we will discuss how mass spectrometry (imaging), combined with the use of electron-transfer dissociation (ETD) as fragmentation technique, can be used as a reliable method to identify AMPs in their native cyclic state. Using this approach, we have previously detected and identified human neutrophil peptides (HNPs) as important AMPs in cancer, of which a detailed bacterial, viral and cancer-related overview will be presented.

Keywords: human neutrophil peptide 1, 2 and 3 (HNP1-3), proteomics, mass spectrometry (imaging), immunomodulatory function, non-small cell lung cancer (NSCLC)

1. Introduction

In the beginning of last century, the first antimicrobial protein, lysozyme, was reported. A few years later, the best known antimicrobial compound, called penicillin, was discovered, which made research into natural antimicrobial proteins/peptides (AMPs) a very important research domain for therapeutic molecules that can be used against bacterial infections [1]. AMPs are naturally occurring small proteins (or peptides) in different organisms and are produced by many tissues and different cell types, acting as host defense molecules against bacteria, but with some also showing a fast antifungal, antiviral, antiparasitic and antitumor response [1–3].

The largest part of AMPs consists of antibacterial peptides with an inhibitory activity towards bacteria, both Gram-positive and Gram-negative [2]. Studies have revealed that AMPs exhibit an overall positive charge, allowing electrostatic interactions with negatively charged phospholipid groups in the bacterial membrane.

By this attribute, pores can be formed by AMPs to disrupt the membrane integrity. Some AMPs are able to cross the lipid bilayer, followed by disruption of intracellular functions such as blocking enzyme activity or inhibition of protein synthesis, both resulting in bacterial cell lysis [1]. For this reason, AMPs are often referred to 'natural antibiotics'.

AMP activity is not restricted to antimicrobial mechanisms, also AMP activity against parasites has been observed: a few AMPs are reported as antimalarial peptides and can possibly serve as new future drug targets against the malaria parasite. For example, cecropins have been shown to block the development of oocysts into sporozoites, while dermaseptins (and some derivatives) have been found to be able to permeabilize the host cell membrane [4].

Furthermore, a subset of AMPs have shown antifungal characteristics against some fungi commonly found in food and agriculture, but also against the common *Aspergillus* and *Candida albicans* infections [2]. These antifungal peptides can interact with fungal membranes to form pores, comparable to the AMP mechanism in bacteria, but they can also act by targeting the specific fungus cell wall or by acting as nucleic acid inhibitors through direct binding to nucleic acids [5]. A smaller part of AMPs also exhibit antiviral activity, by acting through different mechanisms. A first mechanism includes inhibition of virus attachment and cell membrane fusion. As an example, during the recent COVID-19 pandemic, the antiviral peptide (AVP) EK1C4 has been found to be very effective against S-mediated membrane fusion of the viral particles, thus inhibiting entry of the virus and thereby infection [6]. Another example of inhibition of virus attachment is demonstrated by dermaseptins, which possibly affect the lipid bilayer to alter the fusogenic properties of herpes simplex virus [7]. The virus for host cell infection can also be impeded by the direct action of certain AMPs, such as indolicidin, against enveloped virions, causing membrane instability by destruction of the virus envelope [8]. Combined, there is great potential for future therapeutic development of AVPs for both prevention as treatment of infection [6]. A small number of AMPs are believed to be active as anticancer peptides (ACP). It has been suggested that they specifically target the membrane of cancer cells through interaction with phospholipids, mainly phosphatidylserine, present at the outer leaflet of the cancer cell membrane in higher amounts compared to normal cells. Moreover, the ACP LTX-315 has demonstrated both cytolytic and immunogenic properties towards cancer cells, as LTX-315 induces tumor antigen and danger-associated molecular patterns (DAMPs) release, triggering an immune response towards the cancer cells [9].

AMPs are considered key components of the innate immune system, as shortly after an infection, these are promptly synthesized to neutralize a wide variety of pathogens, but through another mechanism compared to that of cytokines or phagocytes [10]. High concentrations of AMPs are usually required to exert an optimal pathogen killing activity, but *in vivo*, lower concentrations of AMPs are reported, in this case possibly acting as potent immune regulators, also leading to pathogen killing but rather through an indirect mechanism [11]. Besides permeabilizing lipid membranes and bacterial walls, their primary role as antimicrobicidal agents, other targets of AMPs are thus reported. Recently, some AMPs are found to also modulate immune responses in vertebrates, through chemotactic activity, attraction, activation and differentiation of leukocytes and monocytes, influencing Toll-like receptor (TLR) recognition and through secretion of proinflammatory cytokines and chemokines, although their underlying mechanisms have not been fully characterized yet [1].

The best studied AMPs include the human defensins and cathelicidins and both have been shown to be chemotactic: β defensins (hBD) recruit (memory) T cells and immature dendritic cells through their chemotactic activity, suggesting they promote cellular immune responses via interactions with the G protein-coupled receptor CCR6 [11]. Another example of direct AMP chemotaxis includes cathelicidin LL-37, an AMP that has been proven to be chemotactic for neutrophils, monocytes and T cells, but not dendritic cells [11]. Additionally, an indirect chemotactic effect is possible by AMPs through inducing the release of pro-inflammatory cytokines and chemokines, to further refine and activate the innate, and eventually the adaptive, immune response [1, 11]. In synergy with particular immune mediators, LL-37 has been shown to enhance IL-6 and IL-10 cytokine production, even as the production of macrophage chemoattractant proteins (MCP-1 and MCP-3) chemokines, resulting in an strengthened (innate) immune response [12]. Toll-like receptors (TLR) are key players in innate immunity by recognizing microbe-associated molecular patterns (MAMPs). TLR activation leads to secretion of AMPs, but some AMPs, including cathelicidins, can modulate TLR-mediated inflammatory responses by strongly reducing LPS-induced TLR activation, mostly by inhibiting TLR4 [11, 13]. Lastly, AMPs, e.g. cathelicidins and β defensins, also exert a regenerative function by affecting wound healing, by stimulating migration, proliferation and tube formation of endothelial cells, through a cascade of activated pathways [11].

Overall, AMPs are important key players in host protection. Due to increasing antibiotic resistance, several AMPs have good potential therapeutic purposes, ranging from antimicrobial, anti-inflammatory and immunomodulatory properties. Also co-administration of AMPs with existing therapies can have good clinical outcomes [14]. Recently, the ACP LTX-315 which has been described earlier, demonstrated in phase I human clinical studies to be an effective drug, due to its immunostimulatory effect resulting in tumor necrosis [9]. Currently, a phase I clinical trial for transdermally accessible tumors is ongoing to evaluate the efficacy of LTX-315 monotherapy or in combination with immune checkpoint inhibitor immunotherapy [9]. Still, some limitations for the therapeutic use of AMPs need to be resolved: high proteolytic degradation of AMPs (i.e. susceptibility to proteases) is commonly observed, unpredicted toxicity is known to occur, chemical synthesis is costly and delivery of AMP targets to the site of infection can be very difficult [9, 14, 15]. As an example, LL-37 has proven to be very effective against Ebola virus infection, but its use as therapeutic molecule is limited as LL-37 is rapidly degraded and can lose its activity under certain conditions. These limitations were overcome with the design of an engineered LL-37 which prevents cell entry of the virus. The therapeutic outcome of these AMPs in animal models is ongoing, possibly combined with other small molecules that interfere with viral replication or together with virus-neutralizing antibodies [16].

AMPs mostly consist of 10 to 60 amino acids, including mainly basic and hydrophobic residues, resulting in positively charged molecules [1, 2]. They can be classified, based on their structure, into four categories; 1) linear extension structure, 2) α-helical AMPs, 3) AMPs consisting of β-strands stabilized by disulfide bonds and 4) both α-helical and β-sheet structures [2]. Due to their cationic properties, AMPs are easily detectable by mass spectrometric analysis. In addition, structural information of AMPs can be obtained by tandem mass spectrometry in which fragmentation spectra are obtained. Based upon this, the corresponding amino acid sequence can be determined and the precursor ion can be identified [17]. Even if the AMPs have a cyclic nature, due to their cysteine bond formation, mass spectrometry can be used as an identification tool, although a specific approach is needed [18–21]. The added benefit of using proteomic approaches to study AMPs is the fact that the majority of AMPs are post- or co-translational proteolytically processed from their large polyprotein precursor, resulting in the release of the active AMP. This is important as it allows for the identification of the active AMP in physiological conditions. It overcomes the limitations of a genomics approach, as it can be complicated to predict the configuration of the exact active peptide from genomic sequences alone [22, 23]. In addition, due to their high positive charge, distribution of the AMP in a tissue can be analyzed using mass spectrometry imaging (MSI). MALDI MSI is a multiplexed analysis that allows the screening of hundreds of analytes simultaneously in a single tissue section without *a priori* knowledge of the present biomolecules [24–26]. Using MSI, a mass spectrum on every pixel of the tissue is recorded, representing all measured analytes by their mass-to-charge (m/z) ratio. The thousands of generated mass spectra can be combined. This thus provides not only structural information about the AMP, it also retains its spatial distribution and information on the relative abundance throughout the tissue [27]. This can overcome the limitation of antibody-related visualization with AMP-specific antibodies that are in some cases designed towards the non-active part of the AMP.

Overall, mass spectrometry (imaging) is an useful approach for the detection and identification of AMPs in their native and active form.

2. Mass spectrometric detection and identification of human neutrophil peptides 1: 3 (HNP1-3)

2.1 Detection of AMPs in their native state

In the search for positive response patterns towards immune checkpoint inhibitors in non-small cell lung cancer (NSCLC) patients, we recently applied matrix-assisted laser desorption/ionization (MALDI) mass spectrometry imaging (MSI) on pretreatment tumor tissue biopsies. Since no prior knowledge of the molecules is required for MSI analysis, new unknown response patterns and biomarkers can be revealed. An additional advantage of using this visualization technique is that new, unknown biomolecules can be detected in their active and native state.

Using this approach, three peptides *m/z* 3369.5, *m/z* 3440.6 and *m/z* 3484.6 have found to be discriminative between a responding and a nonresponding NSCLC patient towards anti-PD-(L)1 immunotherapy, shown in **Figure 1** [21].

2.2 Identification of (cyclic) AMPs

A major bottleneck of the direct analysis of tissues with MALDI-based MSI is the lack of a reliable identification of the visualized molecules, but it has been proven earlier that peptide/protein identification can be performed by using top-down proteomics. This is a major challenge for identification of cyclic proteins or peptides, due to their intramolecular cysteine bridges.

Mass spectrometry followed by *de novo* sequencing has been described as a highly sensitive analytical technique to detect and characterize AMPs that are present in low concentrations within different species. Structural information of the intact AMP can be obtained by tandem mass spectrometry in which peptide ions are dissociated, resulting in a MS/MS spectrum from which the amino acid sequence can be derived. If required, the identification can be confirmed by comparing MS/MS spectra with those of the corresponding synthetic AMP [28]. Shotgun proteomics was performed on both short- and medium-sized antimicrobial peptides, generated by simulated gastrointestinal digestion, from yellowfin tuna samples. This has led to the identification of in total 572 sequences, followed by subjection to antimicrobial activity assays to unravel their AMP properties to evaluate their possible use as new future antimicrobial drugs [29]. In another study, antimicrobial proteins and peptides were extracted from different parts

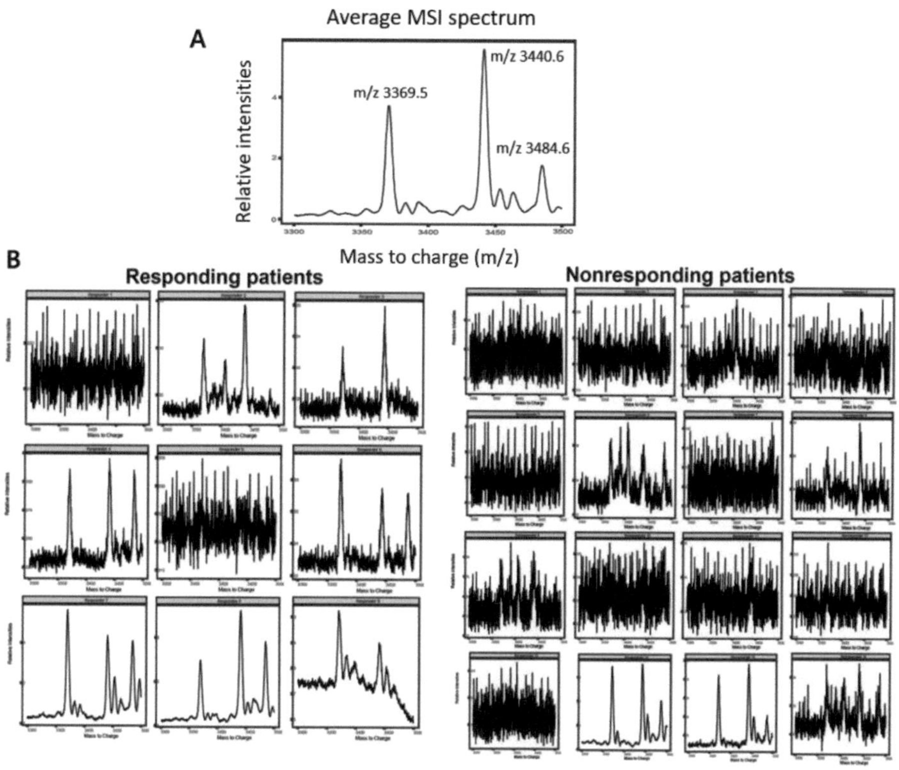

Figure 1.
Average MALDI MSI spectra obtained with mass spectrometry imaging (MSI) analysis of whole formalin-fixed paraffin-embedded (FFPE) tumor biopsies of NSCLC patients. (A) an example of a resulting average mass spectrum with three peptides m/z 3369.5, m/z 3440.6 and m/z 3484.6 of interest. (B) Average MSI spectra of 25 pretreatment tumor FFPE biopsies from NSCLC patients that received anti-PD-(L)1 immunotherapy. From this small patient cohort, nine patients received clinical benefit from the therapy (responders), from which seven patients showed expression of the three interesting peptides. The other 16 NSCLC patients did not derive any clinical benefit from immunotherapy treatment (non-responders), from which 14 show no (or very low) peptide expression. From the nonresponding patients, two NSCLC patients showed interesting peptide expression. Figure adapted from [21] with permission.

of *Charybdis pancration*, a plant used in traditional medicine. These extracts are subsequently tested for their AMP activity against different antibiotic-resistant pathogenic strains. The extracted fraction that has displayed AMP activity, was further analyzed by using mass spectrometry leading to the discovery and identification of seventeen novel peptides with AMP activity [30].

Identification of the cyclic peptides (shown in **Figure 1**) by collision-induced dissociation (either with CID or HCD), a routine approach in top-down peptidome analysis, is mostly not successful as fragmentation of the peptide backbone will not result in multiple fragments of different lengths. Rather, a long fragment with a mass close to the mass of the original parent (minus the loss of H_2O) will be generated, irrespective of where the fragmentation occurred. Hence, these MS/MS spectra cannot be used to deduce a sequence tag that can be used to identify the peptide [31]. However, it has been shown that electron-transfer dissociation (ETD) can be used successfully for the identification of naturally occurring peptides [32], so, ETD has been applied as a fragmentation technique instead of HCD. Rather than generating fragments of the peptides by colliding them with an inert gas in CID, ETD induces fragmentation of large, multiply-charged cations by transferring electrons to them. ETD can be used effectively not only to break the peptide backbone (typically into C and Z ions), but also to reduce any cysteine bridges in the peptide [18–20]. This is nicely demonstrated in **Figure 2B**. An extract of the NSCLC tissue was prepared and analyzed with LC–MS/MS on a LTQ Velos Orbitrap (Thermo Fisher, Waltham, MA, USA) equipped with ETD. This type of instrument combines a dual stage linear ion trap with an orbitrap analyzer, an HCD cell and an ETD source. This allows for a very flexible use of different fragmentation techniques in the ion trap. In this case, the peptide is fragmented by using ETD and the resulting fragments were measured in the Orbitrap. The fragmentation of any of the three target peptides showed a neutral loss of 3 Da in each peptide (**Figure 2B**), corresponding to a reduction of three disulfide bridges between 6 cysteine residues [21].

The reduction of the disulfide bonds in effect turns the circular peptide into a linear one (**Figure 2A** and **B**). In a subsequent experiment, the resulting reduced and thus no longer circular peptide is selected and trapped in the ion trap for an additional fragmentation with CID (**Figure 2C**). In this way, multiple fragments are generated, measured this time in the ion trap, from which an amino acid sequence can be deduced. This leads to the identification of the peptide with mass 3440.6 as human neutrophil peptide 1 (HNP1), presented in **Figure 2D**. The two other peptides of interest were analyzed in a similar way and identified as human neutrophil peptides 2 and 3. These three peptides have an almost identical amino acid sequence, only differing in the first amino acid residue [21].

To conclude, the combined approach of MSI and top-down proteomics using both ETD and CID has revealed human neutrophil peptide 1, 2 and 3, also known as neutrophil defensin 1, 2 and 3, as putative discriminative markers between a responding and a nonresponding NSCLC patient towards immunotherapy [21], highlighting a possible broader role for these AMPs than just a function as

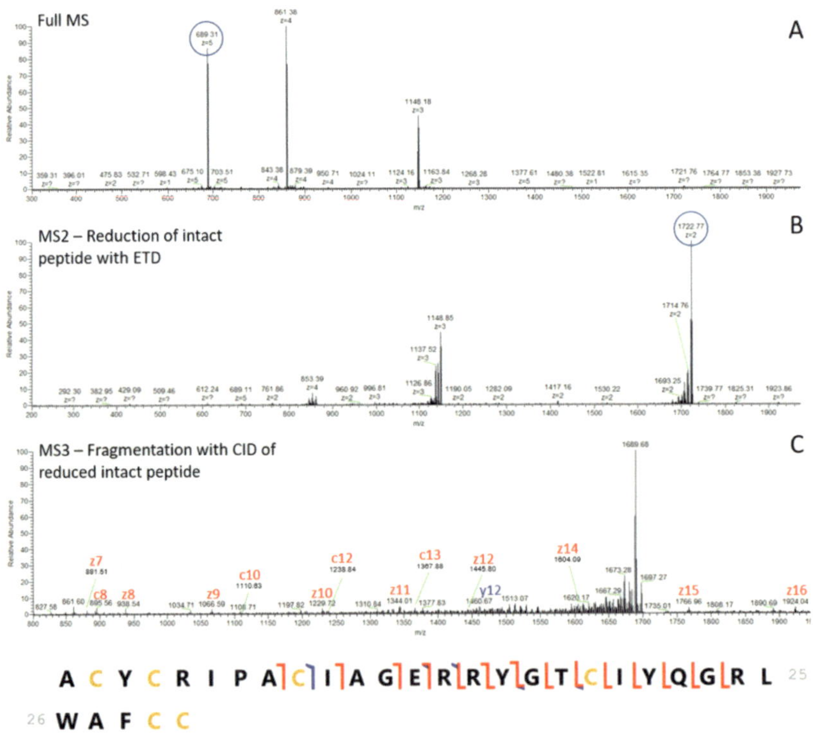

Figure 2.
Mass spectra and annotated sequence of synthetic peptide corresponding for human neutrophil peptide 1 (HNP1). A) Full MS spectrum of intact HNP1, in three different charge states. The five charged ion with m/z 689.31 (mass 3441.6 Da) is selected for reduction of the three internal disulfide bridges with ETD; B) the resulting intact peptide m/z 1722.77 after reduction of three disulfide bridges. This reduced peptide is immediately selected for fragmentation with CID; C) the resulting fragmentation spectrum with c, y and z type ions; D) annotated sequence of human neutrophil peptide 1. Figure adapted from [21] with permission.

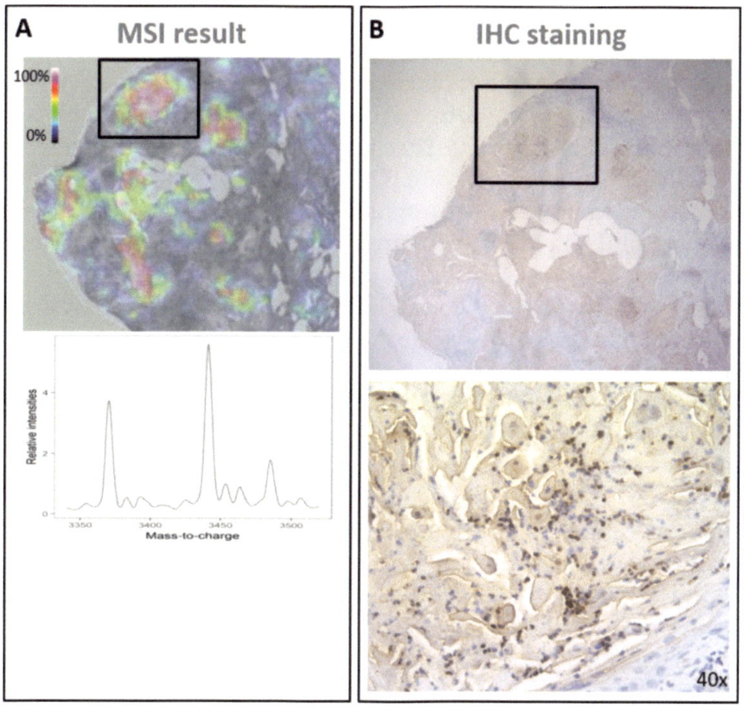

Figure 3.
Distribution of human neutrophil peptides 1-3 in FFPE tissues after MSI and IHC analyses. A) Distribution of HNP1-3 obtained with MSI and the corresponding mass spectrum; B) validation of the presence of HNP1-3 in the same FFPE tissue, prior MSI analyzed, with IHC. The region indicated with the box in the MSI result was compared with the same tissue region after IHC analysis with a defensin 1/3 antibody. Figure adapted from [21] with permission.

antimicrobial peptides. Additionally, these results were verified with immunohistochemical (IHC) analyses on the same pretreatment biopsies with a defensin 1/3 polyclonal antibody. In **Figure 3**, it is illustrated that IHC is feasible on FFPE tissue sections, previously MSI analyzed, without an apparent change in staining intensity [21].

This combined approach has been proven to be very useful in the detection and identification of interesting AMPs, especially in their native, processed form in a clinical context [21].

2.3 The biological activity of HNPs

The previously described observations were a starting point to explore the possible role of neutrophil defensins in cancer immunology.

Defensins, together with cathelicidins, are widely studied, as they were early recognized as important components of the antimicrobial mechanisms of leukocytes. The defensins can be classified in human α-defensins, which are composed of β-strands, and human β-defensins, consisting of both α-helical and β-strands structures [33]. The sequences of these two defensin types include six cysteine residues and their cyclic structure is stabilized by formation of three intramolecular disulfide bonds, from which the cysteine bonding pattern makes a differentiation between α-defensins and β-defensins [33]. These cysteine residues are of major importance for their cationic antimicrobial characteristics [22]. A third class of defensins is also reported, called θ-defensins, and although mRNA expression of θ-defensins has been observed in humans, no functional AMPs from the θ-defensin family are reported to be produced in humans [22].

Currently, 31 β-defensins have been identified and are being studied. They are mainly expressed by epithelial cells and keratinocytes, but can also be secreted from macrophages, neutrophils and lymphocytes, suggesting a broader role in immune responses besides antimicrobial activity [22]. More importantly for this review part are the α-defensin family, more specifically the human neutrophil peptides 1, 2 and 3 (HNP1-3), as previously described. As the name suggests, these AMPs are predominantly produced by neutrophils, but they have also been detected in macrophages, natural killer (NK) cells, immature monocyte-derived dendritic cells and some classes of T and B cells. The fourth α-defensin is also found in these cell types, while α-defensins 5 (HD5) and 6 (HD6) are secreted by intestinal Paneth cells, with the main function to provide intestinal host defense towards pathogens and to control and maintain homeostasis of the intestinal microbiome [22, 34]. HD5 and HD6 deficiency is associated with Crohn's disease, possibly due to the reduced antimicrobial defense capacity by lower HD5 and HD6 expression, leading to an altered microbiome composition [1, 35].

HNP1-3 have an almost identical amino acid sequence, only differing in a single amino acid residue, while this does not hold true for HNP4, HD5 and HD6 (**Figure 4**), although all six α-defensins are characterized by the same cysteine residues [36]. HNP1 and HNP2 (the same is true for HNP2 and HNP3) are released from the same precursor, which is cleaved by a signal peptidase at position 19 leaving a propeptide, which will be further processed by proteolysis in the developing granulocyte. The resulting mature peptide is then packaged into azurophilic granules of the neutrophils, with the HNPs representing more than 30% of the total protein content in these granules [37]. Neutrophils are first-line defense immune cells against different pathogens and are directly recruited to sites of infection, followed by engulfment of the pathogen. Upon neutrophil activation, degranulation of azurophilic granules takes place, thus leading to abundant HNP release as a first-line of response to invading organisms [37–39]. These HNP1-3 have been shown to have antibacterial, antiviral, anticancer and even immunomodulatory activities, which will be discussed further in more detail.

2.3.1 Antibacterial and antiviral activity of HNP1-3

HNP1-3 have a well described antibacterial activity, with demonstrated effectivity towards *S. aureus*, *E. coli*, *P. aerugnosa* and *C. albicans* through interaction of the positively charged HNPs with the anionic bacterial membrane. This can lead to different possible mechanisms, depending on the type of bacterium itself: the most common mechanism of HNPs includes destruction of the bacterial membrane, which is the case for *P. aerugnosa* and *C. albicans.* Lipid II, a bacterial wall precursor, is also a target for HNPs. Such example has been observed in *S. aureus*, in which HNP is responsible for lipid II restriction. In the case of *E. coli,* the disruption by HNP1 happens through intracellular targeting, by inhibiting the bacterium's protein

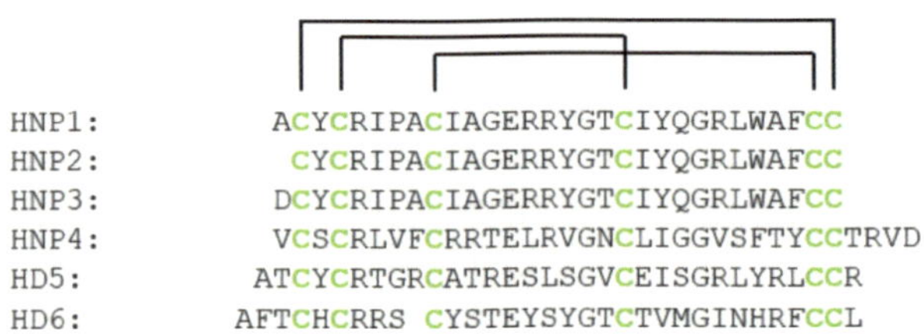

Figure 4.
Alignment of the amino acid sequences of all 6 human α defensins. Conserved cysteine residues are presented in green and their corresponding cysteine bonding pattern is indicated.

synthesis [40]. Furthermore, HNP1 has demonstrated direct activity towards *Mycobacterium tuberculosis*, the pathogen that can cause the infectious disease of tuberculosis, responsible for over a million deaths per year. The direct killing capacity of HNP1 includes permeabilization of the membrane, followed by pore formation [41]. HNP1 has even been considered as a lead compound in combating methicillin-resistant strains of *Staphylococcus aureus* (MRSA). When applied together with antibiotics, the HNPs show a synergistic effect towards different MRSA isolates, paving the way for a new therapeutic approach to overcome the increasing antibiotic resistance [42].

HNP1-3 have not only proven an effective response towards both Gram-positive and Gram-negative bacteria, but antiviral activity is also a well-known characteristic of HNPs, including human immunodeficiency virus (HIV), human papilloma virus (HPV), herpes virus and influenza A virus (IAV) [2]. These HNPs have also been reported as anti-HIV peptides: high production of HNP1-3 by immature dendritic cells have a host protective role against progression of HIV-1, due to the direct HNP damage capability towards the virions, followed by the virion internalization by the immature dendritic cell, leading to viral processing and presentation to HIV-specific CD4+ T cells [43]. In addition, HNP1-3 are identified in the female genital tract acting as host defense forming a natural barrier to HPV [44]. HNP1-3 can inhibit herpes simplex virus (HSV) entry by directly binding to its target receptor and these defensins even exhibit post entry antiviral activity, leading to reduced viral replication after HSV infection [22]. As a last example worth mentioning, these HNPs have an anti-IAV activity by direct interaction with the virus, leading to destabilization of the viral envelope and thus leading to virus inactivation. HNP1 has also been suggested to bind the protein kinase C (PKC) receptor, in this way avoiding both IAV entry and replication [45, 46].

2.3.2 The role of HNP1-3 in cancer (immunity)

Already a direct antitumor effect has been described for human neutrophil peptides in a variety of tumor cells [47]. Furthermore, HNP1 has been reported as a potential prognostic biomarker in cancer [48–50]. In addition, the HNPs are suggested to induce tumor necrosis [48, 49]. Although, despite the reported anticancer activity, defensins HD5 and HD6 are known markers of development and contribution to colorectal tumor growth [51].

In the same study in which we showed an association of the presence of HNPs and a response towards anti-PD-(L)1 immunotherapy in NSCLC, a possible immune stimulatory effect of HNPs towards lung cancer cells has been reported, while no such activity could be shown against non-tumoral cells [21]. *In vitro* data revealed that NSCLC cell proliferation is significantly reduced when cocultured with peripheral blood mononuclear cells (PBMC) from healthy donors. A conceivable explanation for this observation is immune activation towards cancer cells, as an effect of addition of HNPs to the cancer cells was only observed in the presence of PBMC. Direct addition of HNPs to the three NSCLC cell lines in the absence of immune cells did not result in a significant decrease of tumor cell proliferation, and even an increase in tumor cell proliferation was observed in a certain case [21]. Furthermore, IFN-γ secretion was clearly increased in the PBMC and tumor cocultures after HNP-treatment. Surprisingly, treatment of HNPs to PBMC from healthy donors in the absence of NSCLC cells did not result in an increase of IFN-γ release, indicating that HNPs contribute to activate the immune response, although not directly activating the immune cells. Also, non-tumoral cells remain insensitive to the action of HNPs. Neither was the effect explained by treatment with HNPs on the NSCLC tumor cells directly, as HNP treatment of only A549 cells did not result in IFN-γ release [21].

Although earlier studies suggest a direct cytotoxic anticancer activity of the human neutrophil peptides [47–49], in this study, a possible immune–stimulatory effect of HNP1-3 towards lung cancer is suggested. The question raised by these findings is how these HNPs can act as immune-stimulatory effector, not directly on tumor cells nor on the immune cells, while leaving non-tumoral cells intact. A hypothesis is that α-defensins specifically target tumor cells by interaction with phosphatidylserine (PS) exposure. This interaction has been shown in a recent *in vivo Drosophila* model [52]. In general, cell membranes consist of PS that normally faces the inside of the cell due to the activity of phospholipid flippases. In apoptotic cells, PS can be exposed to the outer surface of the cells by loss of flippase activity and by activation of scramblases. In Drosophila, externalized PS serves as a marker for engulfment by macrophages leading to phagocytosis [53]. This mechanism seems to be preserved in human cells, including lung cancer cells [54], and cancerous cells often increase exposure of the negatively charged PS on the outer leaflet of the cell membrane [55]. This would allow for the positively charged HNPs to interact with the negatively charged tumor cell surface PS, resulting in their cell death, while healthy cells remain insensitive to the HNP action, as PS is still present on the inner leaflet of the cell membrane by flippase activity [52].

PS exposure by the tumor cells have been driven in *Drosophila* through tumor necrosis factor (TNF) expression, while this exposure has not been observed on the normal cells [52, 54]. TNF-α concentrations have also been measured in the supernatants of the PBMC and tumor cocultures treated with HNP1-3. For the NSCLC cell lines, an increase in TNF-α release was observed when the coculture was HNP treated, which was not observed for solely PBMC cultures nor for human bronchial epithelial cells BEAS-2B cocultured with PBMCs of three healthy donors [17]. This can possibly explain phosphatidylserine exposure on NSCLC cell lines, making the NSCLC cell membrane sensitive for interaction with the positively charged HNP to induce transmembrane permeability, a typical AMP characteristic [1]. In this way, tumor-associated antigens (TAAs) could be exposed to activate cell-mediated immunity by provoking an immunogenic response, resulting in a significant decrease in tumor cell proliferation [17, 21].

It is conceivable that HNPs play an immune-stimulatory role towards (lung) cancer cells. Due to their direct antimicrobial activity characteristics, HNPs are considered to be part of the innate immune response, just as neutrophils, their main cellular source, as approximately 9% of the neutrophil protein content includes HNPs [56]. Neutrophils have Jekyll and Hyde properties in relation to cancer, as they have been shown to elicit both antitumoral as protumoral activities [57, 58]. Tumor-associated neutrophils (TANs) have been linked with poor prognosis in late-stage tumorigenesis [58, 59]. Although, recent findings indicate antitumor properties of neutrophils in early-stage human tumors; neutrophils have been shown to present antigens, resulting in T cell interaction leading to a proper T cell activation and response. Furthermore, neutrophils are able to attract and activate these T cells through cytokine secretion [60]. It has also been proven that HNPs enhances adaptive immunity, however, their mechanisms remain largely unknown. Nevertheless, studies have shown that HNPs have immunostimulatory characteristics through chemoattraction of naïve T cells [61], $CD8^+$ T cells [37], monocytes [37], maturation and differentiation of immature dendritic cells [43, 61] and by inducing pro-inflammatory chemokine and cytokine production, such as IFN-γ, IL-8 and IL-2 [62].

Chemoattraction of monocytes by HNP has been proven by De Yang *et al.* by analyzing interleukin-8 induced neutrophil-derived T cell attraction. HNP selectively attracted CD4+ naïve T cells and cytotoxic CD8+ T cells for an effective immune response, but not memory CD4+ T cells [61]. In addition, HNP promotes an antigen-specific immune response by chemoattracting dendritic cells, the most potent antigen-presenting cells (APCs). When administered together with antigens, HNPs are able to recruit immature dendritic cells and T cells to microbial infection sites, leading to maturation of these monocytes responsible in promoting an adaptive immunity towards microorganisms [61]. It has also been proven *ex vivo* that human monocyte-derived dendritic cells (moDCs) undergo maturation and differentiation as response to HNPs, but the DC maturation procedure remains unknown [56]. This mechanism seems to be HNP dose dependent: high concentrations (micromolar range) of HNP are able to directly disrupt cell membranes of microorganisms or some tumor cells, through formation of pores in the cell membrane or by interacting with negatively charged molecules [61, 63]. Lower concentrations of HNP (nanomolar range) are thought to bind specific cell receptors, responsible for chemotactic activities and thus resulting in a immunostimulatory effect [56, 61].

Monocyte-derived dendritic cells seem to play an important role in this HNP-driven immunity: moDCs can internalize and process antigens in their immature state, followed by maturation of moDCs by upregulating MHC class II molecules that react with naive CD4 and CD8 T cells to induce their activation, leading to induction of adaptive immunity [43, 56]. HNPs are thus thought to form a link between innate and adaptive immunity, by serving as chemoattractants and immune cell activators [37]. It is demonstrated that HNP-driven DC activation leads to an increased DC capacity to stimulate T cells, explaining the possible HNP interplay in adaptive immunity [61, 64, 65]. Also in an *in vitro* cancer-related context, HNPs have been produced at the tumor site and showed to be chemoattracting for moDCs and to promote the production of stimulatory cytokines [65]. In this way, an antitumor immune response can be exerted, as an enhanced antigen presentation is established by the HNP-driven DC maturation. This shows promising potential for the use of HNPs in anticancer therapy [66].

3. Conclusions

During the last decades, it became more clear that antimicrobial peptides (AMPs) are not restricted in characteristics as being antibacterial, but that AMPs are also serving as a first-line of defense against fungi, viruses, and even tumor cells. Furthermore, these small cationic molecules have been shown to exhibit potent immune regulatory activities, including chemoattraction, activation and differentiation of leukocytes and monocytes to initiate and further enhance adaptive immunity. Combined, we believe that AMPs may hold great potential to be used as lead for new (co-)therapeutic agents.

With proteomic approaches, more in particular mass spectrometry, it is feasible to identify (cyclic) AMPs in their active form after their corresponding proteolysis. While emphasis has been put strongly on HNP identification in a tumorimmunology-related context, it is also important to stress out that mass spectrometric analyses allows for the detection and identification of native AMPs in different specimens, even when present at low concentrations. These unbiased analyses can lead to the detection and identification of new AMPs, important for future drug development.

In this way, human neutrophil peptide (HNP) 1, 2 and 3 were identified in a non-small cell lung cancer (NSCLC) related context, of which the presence have been shown to be discriminative between a responding and a nonresponding NSCLC patient towards anti-PD-(L)1 immunotherapeutics. Although the biological activity of HNPs is well described against bacteria and viruses, little is known about their antitumor characteristics. Some studies suggest a direct antitumoral activity of HNP1-3, while it has also been proven that these HNPs do not show a direct cytolytic activity towards NSCLC, but a reduced NSCLC proliferation was observed in the presence of HNP and peripheral blood mononuclear cells (PBMC) *in vitro.* In the latter case, increasement of IFN-γ was observed, referring a cell-mediated immunity. The question raised by these findings is; what is the mechanism of HNP-mediated immunity? Do the HNPs attack the NSCLC cells directly through interaction with the negatively charged phosphatidylserine on the outer leaflet of the tumor cells? This may result in tumor-associated antigen release responsible for activation of a proper immune response. Also, it is increasingly evident that these HNPs are responsible for an enhanced antigen-specific immune response by activating dendritic cells: upon HNP stimulation, dendritic cells are recruited to the tumor site, followed by maturation and differentiation of these dendritic cells, leading to an enhanced adaptive immune response. However, the exact HNP-driven mechanisms are still largely unknown. Further investigation will reveal if HNPs could be a promising approach in future anticancer therapeutics, possibly in synergy with immunotherapy.

Author details

Eline Berghmans[1,2] and Geert Baggerman[1,2]*

1 Centre For Proteomics, University of Antwerp, Antwerp, Belgium

2 Flemish Institute for Technological Research (VITO), Belgium

*Address all correspondence to: geert.baggerman@vito.be

References

[1] Zhang LJ, Gallo RL: Antimicrobial peptides. Curr Biol. 2016; 26: R14–R19. DOI: 10.1016/j.cub.2015.11.017

[2] Huan Y, Kong Q, Mou H, et al.: Antimicrobial Peptides: Classification, Design, Application and Research Progress in Multiple Fields. Front Microbiol. 2020; 11: 1-21. DOI: 10.3389/fmicb.2020.582779

[3] Brogden KA: Antimicrobial peptides: Pore formers or metabolic inhibitors in bacteria? Nat Rev Microbiol. 2005; 3: 238-250. DOI: 10.1038/nrmicro1098

[4] Vale N, Aguiar L, Gomes P: Antimicrobial peptides : a new class of antimalarial drugs? Front Pharmacol. 2014; 5: 1-13. DOI: 10.3389/fphar.2014.00275

[5] De Cesare GB, Cristy SA, Garsin DA, et al.: Antimicrobial peptides: A new frontier in antifungal therapy. MBio. 2020; 11: 1-21. DOI: 10.1128/mBio.02123-20

[6] Xia S, Liu M, Wang C, et al.: Inhibition of SARS-CoV-2 (previously 2019-nCoV) infection by a highly potent pan-coronavirus fusion inhibitor targeting its spike protein that harbors a high capacity to mediate membrane fusion. Cell Res. 2020; 30: 343-355. DOI: 10.1038/s41422-020-0305-x

[7] Belaid A, Aouni M, Khelifa R, et al.: In vitro antiviral activity of dermaseptins against herpes simplex virus type 1. J Med Virol. 2002; 66: 229-234. DOI: 10.1002/jmv.2134

[8] Edward Robinson W, McDougall B, Tran D, et al.: Anti-HIV-1 activity of indolicidin, an antimicrobial peptide from neutrophils. J Leukoc Biol. 1998; 63: 94-100. DOI: 10.1002/jlb.63.1.94

[9] Tornesello AL, Borrelli A, Buonaguro L, et al.: Antimicrobial Peptides as Anticancer Agents: Functional Properties and Biological Activities. Molecules. 2020; 25: 1-25. DOI: 10.3390/molecules25122850

[10] Pasupuleti M, Schmidtchen A, Malmsten M, et al.: Antimicrobial peptides : key components of the innate immune system Antimicrobial peptides : key components of the innate immune system. Crit Rev Biotechnol. 2012; 32: 143-171. DOI: 10.3109/07388551.2011.594423

[11] Lai Y, Gallo RL: AMPed Up immunity: how antimicrobial peptides have multiple roles in immune defense. Trends Immunol. 2009; 30: 131-141. DOI: 10.1016/j.it.2008.12.003.AMPed

[12] Yu J, Mookherjee N, Wee K, et al.: Host Defense Peptide LL-37, in Synergy with Inflammatory Mediator IL-1β, Augments Immune Responses by Multiple Pathways. J Immunol. 2007; 179: 7684-7691. DOI: 10.4049/jimmunol.179.11.7684

[13] Scheenstra MR, van Harten RM, Veldhuizen EJA, et al.: Cathelicidins Modulate TLR-Activation and Inflammation. Front Immunol. 2020; 11: 1-16. DOI: 10.3389/fimmu.2020.01137

[14] Kang HK, Kim C, Seo CH, et al.: The therapeutic applications of antimicrobial peptides (AMPs): a patent review. J Microbiol. 2017; 55: 1-12. DOI: 10.1007/s12275-017-6452-1

[15] Seo MD, Won HS, Kim JH, et al.: Antimicrobial peptides for therapeutic applications: A review. Molecules. 2012; 17: 12276-12286. DOI: 10.3390/molecules171012276

[16] Yu Y, Cooper CL, Wang G, et al.: Engineered Human Cathelicidin Antimicrobial Peptides Inhibit Ebola Virus Infection. iScience. 2020; 23: 100999. DOI: 10.1016/j.isci.2020.100999

[17] Berghmans E. Mass spectrometry imaging combined with top-down proteomics to predict a more accurate immunotherapy response in non-small cell lung cancer patients [thesis]. Antwerpen: Universiteit Antwerpen; 2020.

[18] Cole SR, Ma X, Zhang X, et al.: Electron Transfer Dissociation (ETD) of peptides containing intrachain disulfide bonds. J Am Soc Mass Spectrom. 2012; 23: 310-320. DOI: 10.1007/s13361-011-0300-z

[19] Wu S-L, Jiang H, Lu Q, et al.: Mass Spectrometric Determination of Disulfide Linkages in Recombinant Therapeutic Proteins Using On-line LC-MS with Electron Transfer Dissociation (ETD). Anal Chem. 2009; 81: 112-122. DOI: 10.1007/s10439-011-0452-9.Engineering

[20] Compton PD, Strukl J V., Bai DL, et al.: Optimization of electron transfer dissociation via informed selection of reagents and operating parameters. Anal Chem. 2012; 84: 1781-1785. DOI: 10.1021/ac202807h

[21] Berghmans E, Jacobs J, Deben C, et al.: Mass Spectrometry Imaging Reveals Neutrophil Defensins as Additional Biomarkers for Anti-PD-(L)1 Immunotherapy Response in NSCLC Patients. Cancers (Basel). 2020; 12: 863. DOI: 10.3390/cancers12040863

[22] Ahmed A, Siman-Tov G, Hall G, et al.: Human antimicrobial peptides as therapeutics for viral infections. Viruses. 2019; 11: 1-26. DOI: 10.3390/v11080704

[23] Azkargorta M, Soria J, Ojeda C, et al.: Human basal tear peptidome characterization by CID, HCD, and ETD followed by in silico and in vitro analyses for antimicrobial peptide identification. J Proteome Res. 2015; 14: 2649-2658. DOI: 10.1021/acs.jproteome.5b00179

[24] Chughtai K, Heeren RMA: Mass Spectrometric Imaging for Biomedical Tissue Analysis - Chemical Reviews (ACS Publications). Chem Rev. 2011; 110: 3237-3277. DOI: 10.1021/cr100012c. Mass

[25] Minerva L, Clerens S, Baggerman G, et al.: Direct profiling and identification of peptide expression differences in the pancreas of control and ob/ob mice by imaging mass spectrometry. Proteomics. 2008; 8: 3763-3774. DOI: 10.1002/pmic.200800237

[26] Ahlf Wheatcraft DR, Liu X, Hummon AB: Sample Preparation Strategies for Mass Spectrometry Imaging of 3D Cell Culture Models. J Vis Exp. 2014; 1-7. DOI: 10.3791/52313

[27] Berghmans E, Boonen K, Maes E, et al.: Implementation of Maldi mass spectrometry imaging in cancer proteomics research: Applications and challenges. J Pers Med. 2020; 10: 1-12. DOI: 10.3390/jpm10020054

[28] Stegemann C, Hoffmann R: Sequence Analysis of Antimicrobial Peptides by Tandem Mass Spectrometry. Methods Mol Biol.; 494. DOI: 10.1007/978-1-59745-419-3

[29] Cerrato A, Capriotti AL, Capuano F, et al.: Identification and Antimicrobial Activity of Medium-Sized and Short Peptides from Yellowfin Tuna (*Thunnus albacares*) Simulated Gastrointestinal Digestion. Foods.; 9

[30] Cunsolo V, Schicchi R, Chiaramonte M, et al.: Identification of New Antimicrobial Peptides from Mediterranean Medical Plant Charybdis pancration (Steinh.) Speta. Antibiotics. 2020; 9: 1-13

[31] Berghmans E, Van Raemdonck G, Schildermans K, et al.: MALDI Mass Spectrometry Imaging Linked with Top-Down Proteomics as a Tool to Study the Non-Small-Cell Lung Cancer

Tumor Microenvironment. Methods Protoc. 2019; 2: 1-21. DOI: 10.3390/mps2020044

[32] Sasaki K, Osaki T, Minamino N: Large-scale identification of endogenous secretory peptides using electron transfer dissociation mass spectrometry. Mol Cell Proteomics. 2013; 12: 700-709. DOI: 10.1074/mcp.M112.017400

[33] Andersson DI, Hughes D, Kubicek-Sutherland JZ: Mechanisms and consequences of bacterial resistance to antimicrobial peptides. Drug Resist Updat. 2016; 26: 43-57. DOI: 10.1016/j.drup.2016.04.002

[34] Ehmann D, Wendler J, Koeninger L, et al.: Paneth cell α-defensins HD-5 and HD-6 display differential degradation into active antimicrobial fragments. Proc Natl Acad Sci U S A. 2019; 116: 3746-3751. DOI: 10.1073/pnas.1817376116

[35] Shimizu Y, Nakamura K, Yoshii A, et al.: Paneth cell α-defensin misfolding correlates with dysbiosis and ileitis in Crohn's disease model mice. Life Sci Alliance. 2020; 3: 1-15. DOI: 10.26508/LSA.201900592

[36] Szyk A, Wu Z, Tucker K, et al.: Crystal structures of human α-defensins HNP4, HD5, and HD6. Protein Sci. 2006; 15: 2749-2760. DOI: 10.1110/ps.062336606

[37] Droin N, Hendra JB, Ducoroy P, et al.: Human defensins as cancer biomarkers and antitumour molecules. J Proteomics. 2009; 72: 918-927. DOI: 10.1016/j.jprot.2009.01.002

[38] Beckloff N, Diamond G: Computational Analysis Suggests Beta-Defensins Are Processed to Mature Peptides By Signal Peptidase. Protein Pept Lett. 2008; 15: 536-540. DOI: 10.2174/092986608784567618

[39] Luthfi M, Setijanto D, Rahardjo MB, et al.: Correlation between human neutrophil peptide 1-3 secretion and azurophilic granule (CD63) expression in early childhood caries. 2019; 16: 81-86. DOI: 10.4103/1735-3327.250973

[40] Amerikova M, Pencheva El-Tibi I, Maslarska V, et al.: Antimicrobial activity, mechanism of action, and methods for stabilisation of defensins as new therapeutic agents. Biotechnol Biotechnol Equip. 2019; 33: 671-682. DOI: 10.1080/13102818.2019.1611385

[41] Khusro A, Aarti C, Agastian P: Anti-tubercular peptides: A quest of future therapeutic weapon to combat tuberculosis. Asian Pac J Trop Med. 2016; 9: 1023-1034. DOI: 10.1016/j.apjtm.2016.09.005

[42] Bolatchiev A: Antibacterial activity of human defensins against *Staphylococcus aureus* and *Escherichia coli*. PeerJ.; 8. DOI: 10.7717/peerj.10455

[43] Rodríguez-García M, Climent N, Oliva H, et al.: Increased α-defensins 1-3 production by dendritic cells in HIV-infected individuals is associated with slower disease progression. PLoS One. 2010; 5: e9436. DOI: 10.1371/journal.pone.0009436

[44] Buck CB, Day PM, Thompson CD, et al.: Human α-defensins block papillomavirus infection. Proc Natl Acad Sci U S A. 2006; 103: 1516-1521. DOI: 10.1073/pnas.0508033103

[45] Salvatore M, Garcı A, Ruchala P, et al.: a-Defensin Inhibits Influenza Virus Replication by Cell-Mediated Mechanism(s). 2007; 100129: 835-843. DOI: 10.1086/521027

[46] Hsieh I, Hartshorn KL: The Role of Antimicrobial Peptides in Influenza Virus Infection and Their Potential as Antiviral and Immunomodulatory Therapy. Pharmaceuticals.; 9. DOI: 10.3390/ph9030053

[47] Ferdowsi S, Pourfathollah AA, Amiri F, et al.: Evaluation of anticancer activity of α-defensins purified from neutrophils trapped in leukoreduction filters. Life Sci. 2019; 224: 249-254. DOI: 10.1016/j.lfs.2019.03.072

[48] Gaspar D, Freire JM, Pacheco TR, et al.: Apoptotic human neutrophil peptide-1 anti-tumor activity revealed by cellular biomechanics. Biochim Biophys Acta - Mol Cell Res. 2015; 1853: 308-316. DOI: 10.1016/j.bbamcr.2014.11.006

[49] Müller CA, Markovic-Lipkovski J, Klatt T, et al.: Human α-Defensins HNPs-1, −2, and −3 in Renal Cell Carcinoma. Am J Pathol. 2002; 160: 1311-1324. DOI: 10.1016/S0002-9440(10)62558-8

[50] Bateman A, Singh A, Jothy S, et al.: The levels and biologic action of the human neutrophil granule peptide HP-1 in lung tumors. Peptides. 1992; 13: 133-139. DOI: 10.1016/0196-9781(92)90152-S

[51] Mothes H, Melle C, Ernst G, et al.: Human Neutrophil Peptides 1-3 - Early markers in development of colorectal adenomas and carcinomas. Dis Markers. 2008; 25: 123-129. DOI: 10.1155/2008/693937

[52] Parvy J-P, Yu Y, Dostalova A, et al.: The antimicrobial peptide defensin cooperates with tumour necrosis factor to drive tumour cell death in Drosophila. Elife. 2019; 8: 1-26. DOI: 10.7554/elife.45061

[53] Cory S: Phosphatidylserine hide-and-seek. Proc Natl Acad Sci U S A. 2018; 115: 12092-12094. DOI: 10.1073/pnas.1817485115

[54] Sharma B, Kanwar SS: Phosphatidylserine: A cancer cell targeting biomarker. Semin Cancer Biol. 2018; 52: 17-25. DOI: 10.1016/j.semcancer.2017.08.012

[55] Nguyen VP, Dixson AC, Barrera FN: The effect of phosphatidylserine on the membrane insertion of the cancer-targeting ATRAM peptide is defined by the non-inserting end. BioRxiv. 2019; 1: 1-13. DOI: 10.1017/CBO978110741 5324.004

[56] Rodríguez-garcía M, Oliva H, Climent N, et al.: Impact of α - defensins1 – 3 on the maturation and differentiation of human monocyte-derived DCs. Concentration-dependent opposite dual effects. Clin Immunol. 2009; 131: 374-384. DOI: 10.1016/j.clim.2009.01.012

[57] Huang HW, Charron NE: Understanding membrane-active antimicrobial peptides. Q Rev Biophys. 2017; 50: 1-17. DOI: 10.1017/S0033583517000087

[58] Riedl S, Rinner B, Asslaber M, et al.: In search of a novel target - Phosphatidylserine exposed by non-apoptotic tumor cells and metastases of malignancies with poor treatment efficacy. Biochim Biophys Acta - Biomembr. 2011; 1808: 2638-2645. DOI: 10.1016/j.bbamem.2011.07.026

[59] Rousseau A, McEwen AG, Poussin-Courmontagne P, et al.: TRAF4 Is a Novel Phosphoinositide-Binding Protein Modulating Tight Junctions and Favoring Cell Migration. PLoS Biol.; 11. DOI: 10.1371/journal.pbio.1001726

[60] Granot Z: Neutrophils as a Therapeutic Target in Cancer. Front Immunol. 2019; 10: 1710. DOI: 10.3389/fimmu.2019.01710

[61] Yang D, Chen Q, Chertov O, et al.: Human neutrophil defensins selectively chemoattract naive T and immature dendritic cells brane of microbes. J Leukoc Biol. 2000; 68: 9-14. DOI: 10.1189/jlb.68.1.9

[62] Vaschetto R, Grinstein J, Del Sorbo L, et al.: Role of human

neutrophil peptides in the initial interaction between lung epithelial cells and CD4 + lymphocytes. J Leukoc Biol. 2007; 81: 1022-1031. DOI: 10.1189/jlb.0706435

[63] Ganz T: The Role of Antimicrobial Peptides in Innate Immunity. Integr Comp Biol. 2003; 43: 300-304. DOI: 10.1093/icb/43.2.300

[64] Rodríguez-García M, Oliva H, Climent N, et al.: Human immature monocyte-derived dendritic cells produce and secrete α-defensins 1-3. J Leukoc Biol. 2007; 82: 1143-1146. DOI: 10.1189/jlb.0507295

[65] Presicce P, Giannelli S, Taddeo A, et al.: Human defensins activate monocyte-derived dendritic cells, promote the production of proinflammatory cytokines, and up-regulate the surface expression of CD91. J Leukoc Biol. 2009; 86: 941-948. DOI: 10.1189/jlb.0708412

[66] Wang Y, Li D, Shi H, et al.: Intratumoral Expression of Mature Human Neutrophil Peptide-1 Mediates Antitumor Immunity in Mice. 2009; 15: 6901-6912. DOI: 10.1158/1078-0432.CCR-09-0484

Chapter 7

Cloning and Identification System of *Apis mellifera* Melittin cDNA in *Escherichia coli*

Diego Jáuregui, Miquel Blasco and Santiago Mafla

Abstract

Honey bee venom, known as apitoxin, is composed of several peptides, the most important of which is melittin. This peptide is a current focus of research since it can improve the immune system and act against cancer due to its anti-mutagenic, anti-inflammatory, and even contraceptive effects. This makes it very desirable to obtain melittin-producing bacteria, and for this reason, this study has aimed at the cloning of *Escherichia coli* with the melittin gene from western bee. In order to do this, the total RNA of the western honey bee (*Apis mellifera*) has been extracted, and a reverse transcription polymerase chain reaction (RTPCR) has been carried out, at different annealing temperatures (68.0, 68.2, 68.4, 68.6, 68.8, and 69.0°C) to amplify the melittin cDNA. The annealing temperature of 68.4°C has allowed the highest production. Subsequently, this cDNA has been cloned into the pGEM-T vector, which has transformed *E. coli* JM109. This transformation has been corroborated by the blue/white test mediated by X-gal.

Keywords: *Apis mellifera*, *E. coli*, melittin, expression vector, transformation

1. Introduction

Bee venom is a unique weapon in the primordial animal kingdom in the defense of the colony. This poison is formed by a complex mixture of efficient proteins designed to protect bees against a wide variety of predators [1]. Bee venom is found in the abdominal cavity (inside a gland) and contains at least 18 active components that have a wide variety of pharmaceutical properties such as melittin, apamin, adolapin, mast cell degranulation peptide (MCD), enzymes (such as phospholipase), biologically active amines (histamine and epinephrine), and non-peptidic components [2]. Melittin is the main component in the venom of the western bee representing 50% of the total dry weight of the apitoxin [3, 4].

Melittin is synthesized in the form of a precursor called prepromelittin, which plays a crucial role in the attachment of the growing polypeptide chain to the membrane of the endoplasmic reticulum and its vectorial discharge into the lumen [5]. This is because it contains a signal peptide that could be removed by the enzyme signal peptidase on the luminal side of the endoplasmic reticulum (ER) [6], giving rise to a peptide called promelittin [7].

Prepromelittin was detected upon translation of melittin mRNA in cell-free systems [8], but it has not been found in any cellular system. Promelittin also contains some polar amino acids more than melittin at the N-terminal end that are eliminated by a protease after translation [9]. These polar amino acids at this end ensure that this toxic peptide is never present during its translation into the ribosomes [10]. The main reason for this is that the N-terminal region of melittin is predominantly hydrophobic while the carboxy-terminal region is hydrophilic due to the presence of a stretch of positively charged amino acid [7], leading to an amphipath that allows it to interact with the biological membranes [11]. Melittin has diverse biological and pharmacological activities [12], in particular the ability to modify the functions of the immune system in the body [13]. It has been seen that the addition of melittin to bacteria increases the turgor pressure of the cells followed by a decrease in the cell pressure, which could destroy the cellular envelope and could be the reason for cell lysis and its antimicrobial properties [14]. In human erythrocytes, melittin binds rapidly to its membrane and forms pores leading to an alteration of the permeability that causes the release of hemoglobin to the extracellular medium, and this causes the hemolysis at room temperature [7]. It also has the capacity to affect the dynamics of membrane proteins, causing their aggregation and immobilizing them in the plane of the lipid bilayer [15] and acting as a potent inhibitor of Ca^{2+} ATPase, H^+ K^+ ATPase, Na^+ K^+ ATPase, and protein kinase (**Figure 1**) [7].

Recent experiments have shown beneficial effects in the application of this poison on human health acting as anti-mutagenic, anti-inflammatory, contraceptive, and radioprotectant against cancer [16–18]. Melittin causes the cancer cell death by apoptosis by activating caspases and matrix metalloproteinases [2]. In addition, melittin has a direct suppressive effect in the production of HIV-1 [19]. Due to the multiple therapeutic applications of this oligopeptide, it is desirable to

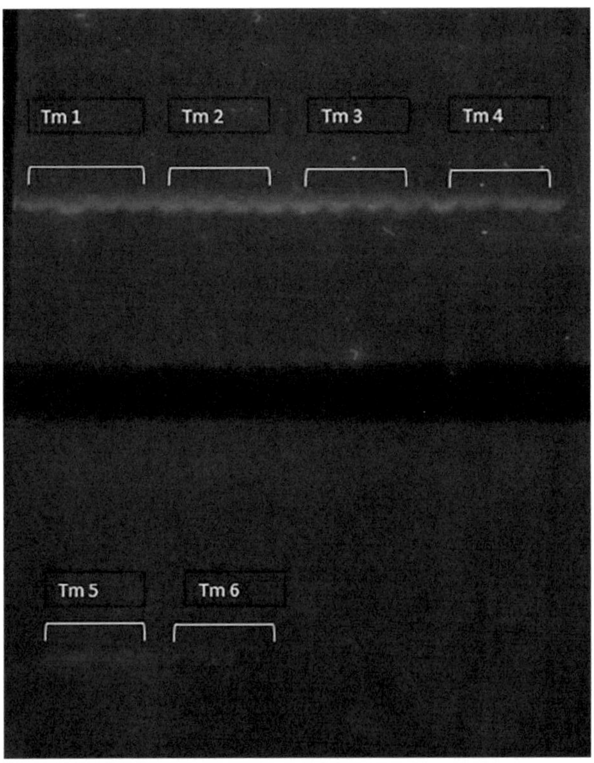

Figure 1.
Electrophoresis gel of PCR from Apis mellifera *melittin at different melting temperatures.*

obtain melittin-producing bacteria for their large-scale production in biological reactors. The objective of this study has been precisely to transform *Escherichia coli* with western honey bee (*A. mellifera*) gene through a plasmidic vector as a first step for an industrial production.

2. Strategies for cloning and expression

2.1 Melittin primers

The preparation of the melittin cDNA primers, both forward and reverse, was carried out first by searching for its sequence in Gen Bank (NCBI), with the accession NC_007073.3. This sequence contains 100 bp and was published by Suchanek et al. [20]. The sequences of restriction sites for ApaLI and SacII were added to the selected primers. Thus, the final sequences of the primers were the following: primer forward 5′TTTTGGGCCCTTAACAGGAAGGA AGGAAGGAA3′ primer reverse 5′AAAACCGCGGAGATCGATAAATCG GCATCG3′.

2.2 RNA extraction

Fifty bees were collected in duly sterilized glass bottles and frozen at −30°C for 30 min in order to conserve the genetic material. The PureYield ™ RNA Midiprep System RNA extraction kit was used to extract and purify the total RNA. The quantification of total RNA was carried out by using the Quantus™ fluorometer [21]. The retrotranscription to total cDNA was carried out using the PureYield RNA Midiprep System (Promega), adding 5 μl of the total RNA extraction to the reaction mixture obtaining a final volume of 20 μl per tube.

2.3 PCR amplification

The PCR mixture was prepared according to the components and the amounts described briefly: a volume (μl) of nuclease-free water 13.25 μl; 5× GoTaq® flexi reaction buffer 5.00 μl; 25 mM $MgCl_2$ 2.00 μl; 10 mM PCR nucleotide mix 0.50 μl; 133.1 pM upstream primer 147.9 pM downstream primer 5 u/μl GoTaq® Flexi DNA polymerase 78 ng/μl cDNA obtained a final volume of 25.0 μl.

The mixture was placed in a thermocycler preheated to 94°C to start the denaturation with for 30 seg. Different temperatures were used for annealing (Tm) in order to determine which of them gave a greater number of copies at the end of the PCR (68.0, 68.2, 68.4, 68.6, 68.8, and 69.0°C; named respectively as Tm1, Tm2, Tm3, Tm4, Tm5, and Tm6) for 60 seg. Finally, the elongation temperature was 72°C for 90 seg, all of them for 40 cycles, and the complete PCR lasted 2 h.

The PCR product was run on 1.5% agarose gel electrophoresis, and the exact amount of cDNA obtained on the most visible band was established by the use of Quantus™ fluorometer (Promega).

2.4 Sequencing

The sample was sent to Macrogen-Korea in order to sequence this amplified fragment by sequencing of new generation. Once the sequence was obtained, it was compared with the melittin accession NC_007073.3 by searching for DNA homologies using the BLAST v1.4 program in GenBank (http://www.ncbi.nlm.nih.gov/BLAST/).

2.5 Insertion of the melittin cDNA in the pGEM-T easy vector

The PCR product was purified using the PCR CleanUp System™ to eliminate primer dimers or other unwanted reaction products in order to improve the ligation efficiency. In order to insert the gene in the vector, 1 µl of the PCR product was taken and mixed with 5 µl of 2× rapid ligation buffer (T4 DNA), 1 µl of pGEM®-T Easy vector (50 ng/µl), 1 µl of T4 DNA ligase (3 µg/µl), and 2 µl of nuclease-free water. These vectors were prepared by cutting with EcoRV and adding a 3'terminal thymidine to both ends. They contain T7 and SP6 RNA polymerase promoters flanking a multiple cloning region within the alpha-peptide coding region of the enzyme beta-galactosidase. Insertional inactivation of the alpha-peptide allows recombinant clones to be directly identified by blue/white screening on indicator plates. The reagents were incubated for 1 h at room temperature. In order to obtain a maximum number of transformants, the reactions were then incubated overnight at 4°C.

2.6 Bacterial transformation

The commercial strain of *E. coli* JM109 was used, maintained at −30°C. Once thawed, 50 µl of this tube was transferred to 1.5 ml microcentrifuge tube, inserted in the ice, and 2 µl of the ligation product was added. The transformed cells were subjected to ice for 2 min, and 950 µl of Super Optimal Broth with Catabolite Repression (SOC) liquid medium [22] at room temperature was added. This solution was incubated for 1.5 h at 37°C with shaking at 150 rpm. Subsequently, aliquots of 100 µl were placed in different plates with Luria-Bertani (LB) semisolid broth medium [23] with 100 µg/ml of ampicillin, 0.5 mM of IPTG, and 80 µg/ml of X-Gal. The plates were incubated overnight at 37°C to perform the Blue-White Screening for positive bacterial transformed colonies/clones.

3. Results

3.1 RT-PCR

It was performed at different annealing temperatures (68.0, 68.2, 68.4, 68.6, 68.8, and 69.0°C). After electrophoresis, it was observed that all the cDNA samples hybridized with the primers obtaining the most visible band at the annealing temperature of 68.4°C. This is, therefore, the hybridization temperature that has resulted in a greater amount of cDNA during PCR. After quantification with the fluorophore, the quantity of cDNA obtained resulted in 78 ng/µl. The PCR product was sequenced prior to cloning by MACROGEN-South Korea.

3.2 BLAST-DNA homology

Searching of the NCBI GenBank database (http://www.ncbi.nlm.nih.gov/) using the melittin accession (Accession no. NC_007073.3) resulted in a similarity index around 80%. The genetic transformation of *E. coli* JM109 with the insert in the vector pGEM-T was corroborated by the blue-white screening test. The colonies formed by nonrecombinant cells therefore appeared blue in color while the recombinant ones appeared white and allowed discrimination between transformants containing recombinant plasmids versus those maintaining self-ligated or uncut vector.

The homology is deduced from the excess of similarity recognized from statistical estimates. A common empirical rule is that two sequences are homologous if they are more than 30% identical over their entire length (much higher identities are seen in short alignments) [24], so it can be firmly stated that both sequences are similar. Due to this, it can be affirmed that *E. coli* has been genetically transformed with the cDNA of western bee melittin. Also, the best annealing temperature has been 68.4°C.

4. Conclusions

Recent studies have highlighted the importance of the melittin as a natural drug for different applications, due to its anti-inflammatory, anti-mutagenic, contraceptive, antimicrobial, and even an anticancer effect. Its mass production is, therefore, of great pharmacological interest and, due to this, obtaining bacteria genetically transformed with this gene becomes very desirable. In other studies, melittin cDNA has been inserted into different plasmids: pBR322 [25], pBV220 [26], and pUC118 [27]. Recently, a gene encoding a hybrid peptide with melittin, called LfcinB (1–15)-Melittin (5–12), has been inserted into the pET-32a vector [28]. In addition, in other study, *E. coli* has been transformed with melittin cDNA from *Apis cerana* [4]. In this work, melittin cDNA from *A. mellifera* has been inserted in *E. coli* using the pGEM-T vector. So, its identification and genetic cloning system have been demonstrated, for its 3'T overhangs at the insertion site, proving a binding successful. Furthermore, the mentioned vector has T7 and SP6 RNA promotors that will ensure its expression in the *E. coli* cells used. Also, another study worked with this vector system [4], suggesting the best way for cloning with these kinds of vectors.

However, it must be remembered that in order to obtain melittin in *E. coli* as a final product, the immature peptide prepromelittin should be posttranslationally modified in some steps. In the first step, the enzyme that catalyzes the hydrolysis of prepromelittin to promilittin is supposed to be widely distributed, since prepromellitin has never been obtained in a cell system. Moreover, promelittin has been obtained in venom glands of honeybees fed with radioactive amino acids [9] and in frog oocytes injected with this mRNA from queen bee [29], but melittin has never been obtained in any tissue that does not come from a species of the genus *Apis*.

For all these reasons, it may be thought the other studies that have cloned melittin cDNA in cell systems that do not belong to species of the genus *Apis*, are likely to give rise to the obtaining of promelittin as a final product, as is the case of the present study. It is necessary to clarify which is the final peptide that has been obtained. If promelittin has been finally obtained, the next focus of study could be to design a protocol to convert it to melittin into *E. coli*.

Acknowledgements

I would like to express my thanks to my patient and supportive, team, who has supported me throughout this research project. I am extremely grateful for our friendly meetings and discussions. I also wish to thank both Universities Ibarra Catholic and Guayaquil, who have been great source of support.

Author details

Diego Jáuregui[1*], Miquel Blasco[2] and Santiago Mafla[1]

1 Departamento de Biotecnología, Pontificia Universidad Católica del Ecuador sede Ibarra, Ibarra, Ecuador

2 Instituto de Investigación e Innovación de Salud Integral, Universidad Católica Santiago de Guayaquil, Guayaquil, Ecuador

*Address all correspondence to: jawy71421@hotmail.com

References

[1] Han S, Lee G. Skin sensitization study of bee venom (*Apis mellifera* L.) in Guinea Pigs. Toxicology. 2002;**28**:1-4. DOI: 10.5487/TR.2012.28.1.001

[2] Oršolić N. Bee venom in cancer therapy. Cancer Metastasis Reviews. 2012;**31**:173-194. DOI: 10.1007/s10555-011-9339-3

[3] Biló BM, Rueff F, Mosbech H, Bonifazi F, Oude-Elberink JNG. Diagnosis of Hymenoptera venom allergy. Allergy. 2005;**60**:1339-1349

[4] Shi W, Xu H, Cheng J, Zhang C. Expression of the melittin gene of Apis cerana cerana in *Escherichia coli*. Protein Expression and Purification. 2004; **37**:213-219. DOI: 0.1006/meth.2001.1262

[5] Suchanek G, Kreil G, Hermodson MA. Amino acid sequence of honeybee prepromelittin synthesized in vitro. Proceedings of the National Academy of Sciences. 1978;**75**:701-704. DOI: 10.1073/pnas.75.2.701

[6] Zimmermann R, Mollay C. Import of honeybee prepromelittin into the endoplasmic reticulum, requirements for membrane insertion, processing and sequestration. The Journal of Biological Chemistry. 1986;**261**:12889-12895

[7] Raghuraman H, Chattopadhyay A. Melittin: A membrane-active peptide with diverse functions. Bioscience Reports. 2007;**27**:189-223. DOI: 10.1007/s10540-006-9030-z

[8] Suchanek G, Kreil G. Translation of melittin messenger RNA in vitro yields a product terminating with glutaminylglycine rather than with glutaminamide. Proceedings of the National Academy of Sciences. 1977;**74**:975-978. DOI: 10.1073/pnas.74.3.975

[9] Kreil G. Biosynthesis of melittin, a toxic peptide from bee venom, amino-acid sequence of the precursor. European Journal of Biochemistry. 1973;**33**:558-566. DOI: 10.1111/j.1432-1033.1973.tb02716.x

[10] Kreil G, Bachmayer H. Biosynthesis of melittin, a toxic peptide from bee venom, detection of a possible precursor. European Journal of Biochemistry. 1971;**20**:344-350. DOI: 10.1111/j.1432-1033.1971.tb01400.x

[11] Huang C, Jin H, Qian Y, Qi S, Luo H, Luo Q, et al. Hybrid melittin cytolytic peptide-driven ultra small lipid nanoparticles block melanoma growth in vivo. Journal of the American Chemical Society. 2013;**7**:5791-5800. DOI: 10.1021/nn400683s

[12] Matysiak J, Schmelzer CE, Neubert RH, Kokot ZJ. Characterization of honeybee venom by MALDI-TOF and nano ESI-Qq TOF mass spectrometry. Journal of Pharmaceutical and Biomedical Analysis. 2010;**54**:273-278. DOI: 10.1016/j.jpba.2010.08.020

[13] Son DJ, Lee JW, Lee YH, Song HS, Lee CK, Hong JT. Therapeutic application of anti-arthritis, pain-releasing and anti-cancer effects of bee venom and its constituent compounds. Pharmacology. 2007;**115**:246-270. DOI: 10.1016/j.phrs.2019.04.002

[14] Mularski A et al. Atomic force microscopy reveals the mechanobiology of lytic peptide action on bacteria. Langmuir. 2015;**31**:6164-6171. DOI: 10.1021/acs.langmuir.5b01011

[15] Husseneder C, Donaldson JR, Foil LD. Genetically engineered yeast expressing a lytic peptide from bee venom (melittin) kills symbiotic protozoa in the gut of formosan subterranean termites. PLoS One.

2016;**11**:1-9. DOI: 10.1371/journal.pone.0151675

[16] Hossen MS, Shapla UM, Gan SH, Khalil MI. Impact of bee venom enzymes on diseases and immune responses. Molecules. 2016;**22**:1-16. DOI: 10.3390/molecules22010025

[17] Perumal-Samy R, Stiles BG, Franco OL, Sethi G, Lim LHK. Animal venoms as antimicrobial agents. Biochemical Pharmacology. 2017;**134**:127-138. DOI: 10.1016/j.bcp.2017.03.005

[18] Rady I, Siddiqui IA, Rady M, Mukhtar H. Melittin, a major peptide component of bee venom and its conjugates in cancer therapy. Cancer Letters. 2017;**402**:16-31. DOI: 10.1016/j.canlet.2017.05.010

[19] Johnston P, Dobson A, Rolff J. Genomic signatures of experimental adaptation to antimicrobial peptides in *Staphylococcus aureus*. G3 Bethesda. 2016;**6**:1535-1539. DOI: 10.1534/g3.115.023622/-/DC1

[20] Suchanek G, Kinas-Mügge G, Kreil G, Schreirer M. Translation of honeybee promelitin messenger RNA, formation of a larger product in mammalian cell-free system. European Journal of Biochemistry. 1975;**60**:309-315. DOI: 10.1111/j.1432-1033.1975.tb21005.x

[21] Díaz C, Garrote H, Amor A, Suárez Y, González R. Cuantificación de ácido ribonucleico para la realización para de la técnica de RT-PCR. Revista Cubana Hematología, Inmunologíay Hemoterapia. 2013;**29**:298-303

[22] Hanahan D. Studies on transformation of *Escherichia coli* with plasmids. Journal of Molecular Biology. 1983;**166**:557-580. DOI: 10.1016/s0022-2836(83)80284-8

[23] Bertani G. Studies on lysogenesis, I, the mode of phage liberation by lysogenic *Escherichia coli*. Journal of Bacteriology. 1985;**62**(3):293-300. DOI: 10.1152/ajpgi.00281.2018

[24] Pearson W. Homology assessment and molecular sequence alignment. Journal of Biomedical Informatics. 2006;**39**:18-33. DOI: 10.1016/j.jbi.2005.11.005

[25] Vlasak R, Unger-Ullmann C, Kreil G, Frischauf AM. Nucleotide sequence of cloned cDNA coding for honeybee prepromelittin. European Journal of Biochemistry. 1983;**135**:123-126. DOI: 10.1111/j.1432-1033.1983.tb07626.x

[26] Zhang Q, Chen Z, Li J, Cai Q, Zhang Q, Zhang F. Cloning of melittin cDNA from honeybee into the high expression plasmid of *Escherichia coli*. Xi Bao Yu Fen Zi Mian Yi Xue Za Zhi. 2004;**20**:406-409. DOI: 10.1111/j.1744-7917.1997.tb00108.x

[27] Wang G, Li D, Fang H. Cloning of promelittin cDNA and its expression in *Escherichia coli*. Wei Sheng Wu Xue Bao. 2001;**41**:181-185

[28] Bi C, Feng X, Shan A, Guo J. Cloning and expression of a gene encoding shortened LfcinB (1-15)-Melittin (5-12) hybrid peptide in *Escherichia coli* BL21(DE3). Sheng Wu Gong Cheng Xue Bao. 2009;**25**:975-981

[29] Kindas-Mugge I, Lane CD, Kreil G. Synthesis and processing of maize storage proteins in *Xenopus laevis* oocytes. Journal of Molecular Biology. 1974;**87**(1):451-462. DOI: 10.1073/pnas.76.12.6448

Chapter 8

Peptides with Therapeutic Potential against *Acinetobacter baumanii* Infections

Karyne Rangel and Salvatore Giovanni De-Simone

Abstract

Antibiotic poly-resistance (multi drug-, extreme-, and pan-drug resistance) is a major global threat to public health. Unfortunately, in 2017, the World Health Organization (WHO) introduced the carbapenemresistant isolates in the priority pathogens list for which new effective antibiotics or new ways of treating the infections caused by them are urgently needed. *Acinetobacter baumannii* is one of the most critical ESKAPE pathogens for which the treatment of resistant isolates have caused severe problems; its clinically significant features include resistance to UV light, drying, disinfectants, and antibiotics. Among the various suggested options, one of the antimicrobial agents with high potential to produce new anti-Acinetobacter drugs is the antimicrobial peptides (AMPs). AMPs are naturally produced by living organisms and protect the host against pathogens as a part of innate immunity. The main mechanisms action of AMPs are the ability to cause cell membrane and cell wall damage, the inhibition of protein synthesis, nucleic acids, and the induction of apoptosis and necrosis. AMPs would be likely among the main anti-*A. baumannii* drugs in the post-antibiotic era. Also, the application of computer science to increase anti-*A. baumannii* activity and reduce toxicity is also being developed.

Keywords: RAMP, *Acinetobacter baumannii*, resistance, action mechanism

1. Introduction

Microbial infections contribute substantially to global mortality trends. Antibiotic resistance is one of the biggest challenges for the clinical sector, industry, environment, and societal development. Unfortunately, the emergence of drug-resistant pathogens is rapidly growing, and the world is heading toward the post-antibiotic era [1, 2]. Bacteria possess three defined types of antimicrobial resistance: intrinsic, acquired, and phenotypic or adaptive resistance [3–11]. Although there are multiple causes of the resistance phenomenon, it is considered that antimicrobial resistance is an old natural phenomenon when microbes are exposed to antimicrobial drugs, with an accelerated evolution triggered not only by the abusive use of antibiotics but also such as wrong choices, inadequate dosing, and poor adherence to treatment guidelines that contribute to the increasing antimicrobial resistance selection [12, 13]. In addition, antibiotic treatment for difficult-to-treat multidrug-resistant bacterial infections is limited [13]. ESKAPE pathogens

(*Enterococcus faecium, Staphylococcus aureus, Klebsiella pneumoniae, A. baumannii, Pseudomonas aeruginosa*, *Enterobacter* species) are among the most common opportunistic pathogens in nosocomial infections [14]. The abbreviation ESKAPE reflects the ability of these organisms to "escape" killing by antibiotics and defy eradication by conventional therapies, which accounts for increased morbidity and mortality for improved resource utilization in healthcare [15]. One of the ESKCAPE pathogens responsible for nosocomial and community-acquired infections is *A. baumannii*, a Gram-negative, non-motile, non-fermentative, and non-sporulated bacterium Moraxellaceae family [16] that is part of the *Acinetobacter calcoaceticus–A. baumannii* complex (Acb). Currently, six species, namely *A. calcoaceticus*, *A. baumannii*, *A. pittii*, *A. nosocomialis*, *A. seifertii*, and *A. lactucae* (a later heterotypic synonym of *A. dijkshoorniae*) [17, 18], belonging to the Acb complex have been associated with human diseases [19]. Even though these species differ in antimicrobial resistance, pathogenicity, and epidemiology [20], the Acb complex is genetically and physiologically highly related, making it difficult to distinguish them phenotypically with standard laboratory methods [21]. Of all the species in the Acb complex, *A. baumannii* is the most widespread in hospitals, even associated with an increased risk of morbidity, mortality, high treatment costs, and long periods of hospitalization [22]. *A. baumannii* causes various infections, including wounds, skin, urinary tract infections, pneumonia, meningitis, and bacteremia [23, 24]. There are several nomenclatures in the literature based on the number of resistance classes of antibiotics. According to Magiorakos et al. (2012), a multidrug-resistant (MDR) strain is resistant to at least one antimicrobial in more than three classes of antimicrobials; and extensively drug-resistant (XDR) strain is one resistant to at least one antimicrobial in all classes of antimicrobials except two or fewer types, and a pan drug-resistant (PDR) strain is resistant to all antimicrobial agents [25]. *A. baumannii* has globally emerged as a highly troublesome nosocomial pathogen revealing MDR, XDR, and PDR phenotypes, and unfortunately, evidence has shown an increased *A. baumannii* antibiotic resistance over time [26]. *A. baumannii* is one of the most critical and fearful pathogens with treatment options limited due to many aspects: its extended virolome and resistome, evasion of the host's immune effectors, ability to survive in extreme environmental conditions, to grow in biofilms, and to switch to latent growth forms with a minimal metabolic rate [27, 28]. The World Health Organization (WHO) has recently published a report, which also highlighted *A. baumannii* resistant to carbapenems (CRAb) [29, 30] which was classified in the group of "priority 1 for research and develop new antibiotic treatments" and was considered as a "critical" pathogen [31]. One of the antimicrobial agents with high potential for research and development of anti-*Acinetobacter* drugs is the antimicrobial peptides [32]. This chapter aimed to review the powerful antimicrobial peptides described with activity against *A. baumannii* multiresistant.

2. Antimicrobial peptides

Antimicrobial peptides (AMPs) may represent an alternative to current antibiotics in MDR *A. baumannii* ESKAPE pathogen [33]. AMPs (also known as host defense peptides) are small polycationic peptides naturally produced by living organisms with both microbicidal and immunomodulatory activities, acting as a primary barrier against pathogens, including protozoa, víruses, bacteria, archaea, fungi, plants, and animals as a part of innate immunity system [34–41]. However, the computational design of synthetic AMPs with improved activity is also being developed [42]. They interact with cell membrane through electrostatic interactions, causing the inhibition of protein and nucleic acid synthesis and final cellular lysis by apoptosis and necrosis [43–44]. In addition to the antimicrobial properties, some AMPs have other activities, such as anticancer antioxidant, wound healing, immunoregulatory [38, 45, 46]. AMPs also play an essential role in regulating immune processes such as activating and recruiting immune system cells, angiogenesis, and inflammation [47]. AMPs are amphipathic molecules with a positive electric charge, varying molecular weight, and containing about 11–50 amino acid residues [47, 48]. AMPs are classified into α-helical, β-sheet, and extended peptide families [49–51] and interact with the membranes initially through electrostatic and hydrophobic interactions (**Figure 1**), accumulating at the surface and self-assemble on the bacterial membrane after reaching a particular concentration [52, 53].

At this stage, various models have been proposed to describe the action of AMPs. The models can be classified under two broad categories: transmembrane pore (TMP) and non-pore models (NPM), and the TMP can be further subdivided into the barrel-stave pore and toroidal pore models. In the barrel-stave model, the AMPs are initially oriented parallel to the membrane but eventually insert perpendicularly in the lipid bilayer [54] (**Figure 2A**), thus promoting lateral peptide-peptide interactions, like that of membrane protein ion channels. Peptide amphipathic structure (α and/or β sheet) is essential in this pore formation mechanism as the hydrophobic regions interact with the membrane lipids and hydrophilic residues from the lumen of the channels [55, 56]. A unique property associated with AMPs in this category is a minimum length of ~22 residues (α helical) or ~ 8 residues (β sheet) to span the lipid bilayer. Only a few AMPs, such as alamethicin [57], pardaxin [58, 59], and protegrins [55], have been shown to form barrel stave channels.

Furthermore, in the toroidal pore model, the peptides also insert perpendicularly in the lipid bilayer, but specific peptide-peptide interactions are not present [57]. Instead, the peptides induce a local curvature of the lipid bilayer with the pores partly formed by peptides and partly by the phospholipid head group (**Figure 2B**). Thus, the dynamic and transient lipid-peptide supramolecule is known as the "toroidal pore." The distinguishing feature of this model compared to the barrel-stave pore is the net arrangement of the bilayer. In the barrel-stave pore, the hydrophobic and hydrophilic sequence of the lipids is maintained, whereas, in toroidal pores, the hydrophobic and hydrophilic arrangement of the bilayer is

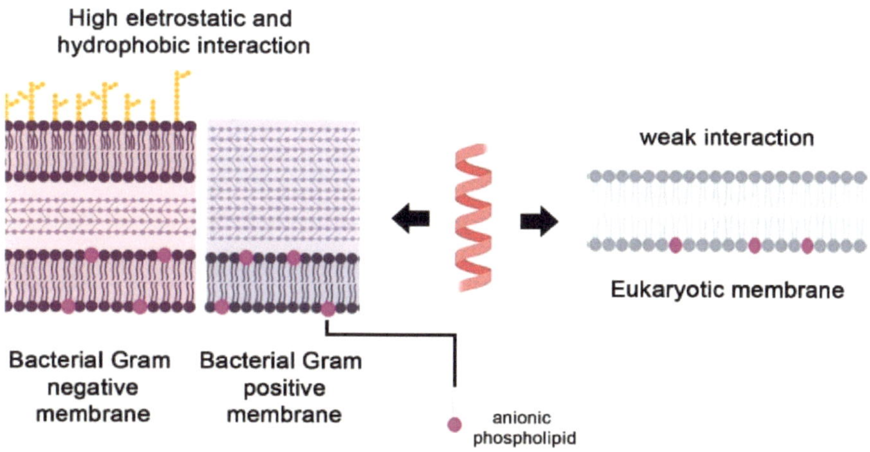

Figure 1.
Interaction of cationic AMPs with eukaryotic and bacterial membranes. Images were created using BioRender.com.

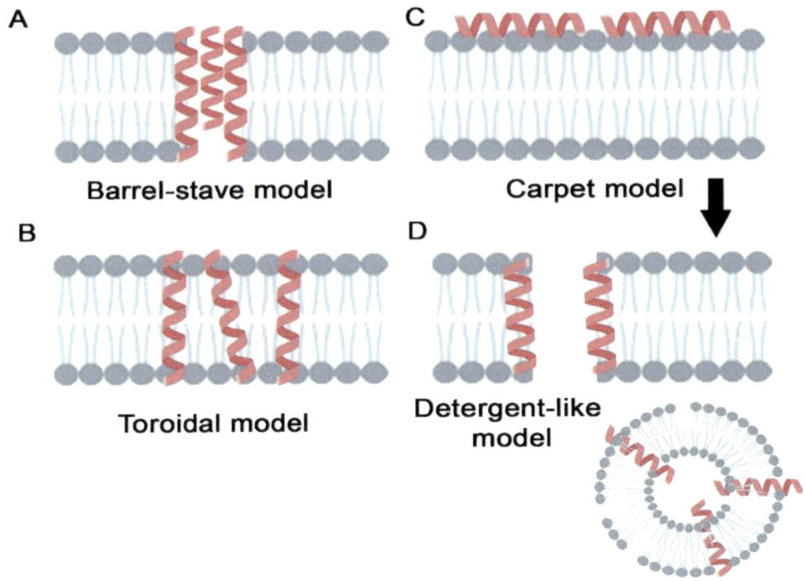

Figure 2.
Mechanisms of action of AMPs in bacteria. A) Barrel-stave model: AMPs stack into the bilayer of the cell membrane to form a channel. (B) Toroidal pore model: Accumulation of vertically and bend embedded AMPs in the cell membrane to form a pore structure, (C) carpet model: Distribution of AMPs on membrane surface that evolve to detergent-like mode, forming micelles, (D) images were created using BioRender.com.

disrupted, thus providing alternate surfaces for the lipid tail and the lipid head group to interact with. Furthermore, as the pores are transient upon disintegration, some peptides translocate to the inner cytoplasmic leaflet entering the cytoplasm and potentially targeting intracellular components [60]. Other features of the toroidal pore include ion selectivity and discrete size [61]. Several AMPs such as magainin 2 [62], lacticin Q [62], aurein 2.2 [63], and melittin [57, 62] have been shown to form toroidal pores. In addition, the type of pore started by aurein 2.2 has been shown to depend on the lipid composition: In a 1-palmitoyl-2-oleoyl-*sn*-glycero-3-phosphocholine (POPC)/1-palmitoyl-2-oleoyl-*sn*-glycerol-3-phospho-(1′-*rac*-glycerol) POPG (1:1) membrane model, the peptides induce toroidal pores, whereas in a 1,2-dimyristoyl-*sn*-glycerol-3-phosphocholine (DMPC)/1,2-dimyristoyl-*sn*-glycero-3-phospho-(1′-*rac*-glycerol) DMPG (1,1) membrane model, the peptides work in a detergent-like model (details below) indicating the importance of the hydrophobic thickness of the lipid bilayer and the membrane composition [64, 65]. Ultimately, both pore-forming models (toroidal pore and barrel) lead to membrane depolarization and eventually cell death.

AMPs can also act without forming specific pores in the membrane. One of these models is designated as the carpet model [61, 62, 66]. In this case, the AMPs adsorb parallel to the lipid bilayer and reach a threshold concentration to cover the surface of the membrane, thereby forming a "carpet" (**Figure 2C**) and leading to unfavorable interactions on the membrane surface. Consequently, the membrane integrity is lost, producing a detergent-like effect, which eventually disintegrates the membrane by forming micelles. The final collapse of the membrane bilayer structure into micelles is the detergent-like model **(Figure 2D).** The carpet model does not require specific peptide-peptide interactions of the membrane-bound peptide monomers; it also does not require the peptide to insert into the hydrophobic core to form transmembrane channels or specific peptide structures [67]. Many peptides act as antimicrobial agents despite their specific amino acid composition or the length of the sequence. Such AMPs typically act using the carpet model [66] at high concentrations because of their amphiphilic nature. Examples of AMPs acting by the carpet model are cecropin [68], indolicidin [69], aurein 1.2 [67], and LL-37 [66].

Overall, there are many models to describe the MOA of AMPs. In addition to those given above, other related models include the interfacial activity model, the electroporation model, and the Shai-Huang-Matsazuki model [62]. Some models do not make the specific distinctions shown in **Figure 2.** For example, it has been suggested that the carpet-like mechanism is a prerequisite step for the toroidal pore model [62]. Most studies to elucidate the MOA of AMPs involve the use of model membranes. The mode of action of only a few AMPs has been investigated with whole bacterial cells using imaging techniques [70, 71]. Different results may be obtained using other membrane models or assay conditions; for example, more than one MOA is possible for certain AMPs such as BP100 as the peptide-to-lipid ratio changes [72], indicating that the models described here may or may not translate directly to what is occurring in bacteria.

An online antimicrobial peptide database, APD3, list examples of AMPs, including both synthetically synthesized and compounds produced by living organisms [37]. In addition, many AMPs are currently being studied to elucidate their therapeutic efficacy against *A. baumannii* strains (**Table 1**).

2.1 Cathelicidins

Cathelicidins are a group of cationic AMPs (CAMPs) (with more than 30 members) detected in the immune system of some vertebrates that have in their structure two domains involved in antimicrobial activity [145]. Compared with carbapenems (imipenem and meropenem), which are considered the drugs of choice for infections caused by MDR *A. baumannii* (MIC = 16–32 mg/L) [146], these peptides exhibit excellent activity.

2.1.1 LL-37

The most studied member of the cathelicidins family is LL-37 (Human cathelicidin) with an α-helical structure. It is produced by many cell types as a part of innate immunity and exhibits broad-spectrum microbicidal activities against Gram-positive and Gram-negative bacteria by plasma-membrane disruption [147]. Other properties were also described, like immunomodulation properties such as chemoattraction and activation of various immune cells, neutralizing the lipopolysaccharide (LPS), regulating the inflammatory response, wound closure, and chemotaxis [38, 148–151]. Feng et al. Investigated the anti-*A. baumannii* activity of LL-37 and fragments KS-30 and KR-12 against one sensitive and four MDR *A. baumannii* clinical isolates [73]. The minimum inhibitory concentration (MIC) for three pieces of KS-30, KR-20, and KR-12 was 8–16, 16–64, and 128–256 μg/ml, respectively. At the same time, LL-37 inhibited all sensitive and drug-resistant strains at the concentration of 16–32 μg/ml. Furthermore, LL-37 and the fragment KS-30 have been found to significantly inhibited and dispersed the *A. baumannii* biofilm in abiotic surfaces at 32 and 64 μg/ml, respectively [73]. A panel of synthetic peptides based on human LL-37 AMP shows potent microbicidal activity against several ESKAPE pathogens without selecting resistance and can also eliminate persister cells and biofilms of *P. aeruginosa*, *A. baumannii*, and *S. aureus* in the micromolar scale [74]. SAAP-148 is an α-helical AMP, able to suppress MDR *A. baumannii* without causing resistance and prevents biofilm formation. Studies showed that this peptide could inhibit the growth of *A. baumannii* MDR at a concentration of 6 μg/m. Treatment with this peptide (animal model) appointment has been shown to eliminate acute and biofilm-related infections by *A. baumannii* in

Peptide	Ref.	Sequence	Structure	MIC against *A. baumannii* (μg/mL)		Source
				Antibiotic-susceptible	**MDR**	
LL-37	[38, 52]	LLGDFFRKSKEKIGKEFKRIVQRIK DFLRNLVPRTES (37aa)	AH	32	16–32	*H. sapiens*
KR-30	[52]	KSKEKIGKEFKRIVQRIKDFLRNLV PRTES (30aa)	AH	16	8–16	*H. sapiens*
KR-20	KRIVQRIKDFLRNLVPRTES (20aa)	AH	64	16–32		
KS-12	KRIVQRIKDFLR (12aa)	AH	256	64–256		
SAPP-148	[53]	LKRVWKRVFKLLKRYWRQLKKPV R (24aa)	AH	—	6	*H. sapiens*
CATH-BF derivative (Cath-A and OH-	[54]	KFFRKLKKSVKKRAKEFFKKPRVI GVSIPF (30aa)	AH	—	8–32	*Bungarus fasciatus* (Snake venom)
ZY4 cathelicidin-BF-15 derived	[55]	VCKRWKKWKR KWKKWCV-NH_2 (17aa)	Cyclic SH-bridge	—	4.6–9.4	
NA-CATH	[56]	KRFKKFFKKLKNSVKKRAKKFFKK PKVIGVTFPF (34aa)	AH	10	10	*Naja atra* (Snake venom)
OH-CATH30	[57]	KFFKKLKNSVKKRAKKFFKKPRVI GVSIPF (30aa)	AH	10	10	*King cobra* (Snake venon)
DOH-CATH30	(KFFKKLKNSVKKRAKKFFKKPRVI GVSIPF, italics indicate D-amino acids)	AH	—	1.56–12.5		
D-Myrtoxin-Mp 1a (Mp1a)	[58]	IDWKKVDWKKVSKKTCKVMXKA CKEL-NH2 (26aa-aipha chain)				
		LIGLVSKGTCVLXKTVCKKVLKQNH2 (23aa-beta chain)	Helical heterodim	25 nM	—	*Myrmecia pilosula*

Peptide	Ref.	Sequence	Structure	MIC against *A. baumannii* (μg/mL)		Source
				Antibiotic-susceptible	**MDR**	
Venon cocktail proteins	[59]	Cocktail	—	—	50.6% of inhibition at 20 mg/mL of venom	*Leiurus quinquestriatus* (Scorpion venom)
Ranalexin	[60]	LGGLIKIVPAMICAVTKKC (19aa)	AH	—	4–18	*Rana catesbeiana (American bulfrog)*
Danalexin		LGGLIKIVPAMICAVTKKC (19aa)	AH	—	4–16	
LS-sarcotoxin	[61]	GWLKKIGKKIERVGQHTRDATIQ TIGVAQQAANVAATLK-NH2	AH	4	4–8	*Lucilla serricata*
)LS-stomoxyn	GFRKRFNKLVKKVKHTIKETANV SKDVAIVAGSGVAVGAAM-NH2	AH	8	4–16		
Mini-ChBac7.5 Nα	[62]	RRLRPRRPRLPRPRPRPRPRPR (22aa)	AH	—	2 μM	Domestic goat (*Capra hircus*)
Mini-ChBac7.5 Nβ		RRLRPRRPRLPRPRPRPRPRP (21aa)	AH	—	4 μM	
AM-CATH36	[56]	GLFKKLRRKIKKGFKKIFKRLPPIG VGVSIPLAGKR (36aa)	AH	5.2	5.2	*American alligator*
AM-CATH28	KIKKGFKKIFKRLPPIGVGVSIPLA GKR (28aa)	AH	28	10		
AM-CATH21	GLFKKLRRKIKKGFKKIFKRL (21aa)	AH	42	10		
WAM-1	[63, 64]	KRGFGKKLRKRLKKFRNSIK KRLKNFNVVIPIPLPG (36aa)	AH	8.12	4–64	Tammar wallaby (*Macropus eugenii*)
Indolicidin	[65, 66, 68]	LPWKWPWWPWRR-NH(2) (13aa)	Other structure	4	2–64	Cytoplasmic granules of the bovine neutrophils
Bactenecin	[65, 67, 69]	LCRIVVIRVCR (12aa)	B-turn structure Ciclyc	64	—	Bovine neutrophil granules, Caprine

Peptide	Ref.	Sequence	Structure	MIC against *A. baumannii* (μg/mL)		Source
				Antibiotic-susceptible	**MDR**	
Bac5	[62, 70, 71]	RFRPPIRRPPIRPPFNPPFRPPVRPPF RPPFRPPFRPPIGPFP-NH2 (42aa)				
Bac7	[72]	Bac7 N-terminal fragments Bac7(1–16; RRIRPRPPRLPRPRPR), Bac7(1–35; RIRPRPPRLPRPRPRPLPFPRPGP RPIPRPLPFP);Bac7(535;PRPPR LRPRPRPLPFPRPGPRPIPRPLPFP) 59aa				
HNP-1	[65]	ACYCRIPACIAGERRYGTCIYQGRL WAFCC (30aa)	AH	50	—	*H. sapiens* (Polymorphonuclear neutrophil)
HNP-2	[65]	CYCRIPACIAGERRYGTCIYQGR LWAFCC (29aa)	AH	50	—	
HD5d5	[73]	ARARCRRGRAARRRRLRGVCRIR GRLRRLAAR (32aa)	AH	40	40	
CL defensin	[74]	ATCDLFSFQSKWVTPNHAACAAH CTARGNRGGRCKKAVCHCRK (43aa)	AH, antiparallel B-sheet; N-terminal loop	—	—	*Cimex Lectularius (Bedbug)*
HBD-2	[75]	GIGDPVTCLKSGAICHPVFCPRRY KQIGTCGLPGTKCCKKP (41aa)	Beta	3.90–9.35	3.25–4.5	Epithelial lining of respiratory /urinary tracts
HBD-3	[76]	GIINTLQKYYCRVRGGRCAVLSCL PKEEQIGKCSTRGRKCCRRKK (45aa)	AH + B-sheet	4	4	
Magainin-1	[65, 77]	GIGKFLHSAGKFGKAFVGEIMKS (23aa)	AH	—	256	Frog skin peptide
Magainin-2	[65, 77, 78]	GIGKFLHSAKKFGKAFVGEIMNS (23aa)	AH	9.8–64	4.9–64	
Pexiganan	[79–81]	GIGKFLKKAKKFGKAFVKILKK (22aa)	AH	1–8	1–8	Frog skin peptide

Peptide	Ref.	Sequence	Structure	MIC against *A. baumannii* (μg/mL)		Source
				Antibiotic-susceptible	MDR	
Aurein 1,2	[81]	GLFDIIKKIAESF (13aa)	AH	16	—	Frog skin peptide
CAMEL		KWKLFKKIGAVLKVL-NH2 (15aa)	AH	2	—	
Citropin 1.1.		GLFDVIKKVASVIGGL-NH2 (16aa)	AH	16	—	
Omiganan		ILRWPWWPWRRK-NH2 (12aa)	AH	32	—	
r-Omiganan		KRRWPWWPWRLI-NH2 (12aa)	AH	16	—	
Temporin A		FLPLIGRVLSGIL-NH2 (13aa)	AH	128	—	
Brevinina 2 (B2RP)	[82]	GIWDTIKSMGKVFAGKILQNL-NH(2) (21aa)	AH	29	7–13.9	Frog skin peptide
[D4K] B2RP	[83, 84]	GIWKTIKSMGKVFAGKILQNL·NH 2 (21aa)	AH	4–16	4–16	Frog skin peptide
B2RP-Era	[83, 85]	GVIKSVLKGVAKTVALGML·NH2 (19aa)	AH	8–32	8–64	Frog skin peptide
Alytesirin-1c	[86]	GLKEIFKAGLGSLVKGIAAHVASNH2 (23aa)	AH	—	11.3–22.6	Frog skin peptide
[E4k] Alytesirin-1c	[83, 84]	GLKEIFKAGLGSLVKGIAAHVAS·NH2 (23aa)	AH	4–16	4–16	Frog skin peptide
[S7K, G11K] Alytesirrin-2a	[87]	ILGKLLKTAAKLLSNL.NH2 (16aa)	AH	—	8	Frog skin peptide
PGLa-AM1	[83, 88]	GMASKAGSVLGKVAKVALKAAL·NH2 (22aa)	AH	16–128	16–128	Frog skin peptide
CPF-AM1	[83, 89, 90]	GLGSVLGKALKIGANLL(19aa)	AH	16–128	4–128	Frog skin peptide
CPF-B1	[91]	GLGSLLGKAFKIGLKTVGKMMG GAPREQ (28aa)		—	11.4–22.8	Frog skin peptide
CPF-C1	[90]	GFGSLLGKALRLGANVL 917aa)		5	—	Frog skin peptide

Peptide	Ref.	Sequence	Structure	MIC against *A. baumannii* (µg/mL)		Source
				Antibiotic-susceptible	MDR	
[E6k,D9k] Hymenochirin-1B	[92]	LKLSPKTKDTLKKVLKGAIKGAIA IASMA-NH2 (29aa)	AH	—	4.9	Frog skin peptide
Hymenochirin-1 Pa	[93]			—	—	Frog skin peptide
[G4K] XT7	[83, 94]	GLLGPLLKIAAKVGSNLL.NH2 (18aa)	AH	4–32	4–64	Frog skin peptide
Buforin II	[66, 77, 95, 96]	TRSSRAGLQFPVGRVHRLLRK (21aa)	AH	8–19.5	0.25–39	Frog skin peptide
Melittin	[65, 97, 98]	GIGAVLKVLTTGLPALISWIKRKR QQ (26aa)	AH	0.25–4	0.25–25	European honeybee (*Apis mellifera*)
Cecropin A	[65, 99]	KWKLFKKIEKVGQNIRDGIIKAGP AVAVVGQATQIAK (37aa)	AH	32	0.5–32	Cecropia moth (*Hyalophora cecropia*)
BR003-cecropin A	[100]	GGLKKLGKKLEGAGKRVFNAAEK ALPVVAGAKALRK (36aa)		5	5	*Aedes aegypti*
Mdc	[101]	GWLKKIGKKIERVGQHTRDATIQ TIGVAQQANAVAATLKG (40aa)		4	4	Housefly *larvae*
Cecropin P1	[65, 102]	SWLSKTAKKLENSAKKRISEGIAIA IQGGPR (31aa)		1.6	—	Pig (*Ascaris suum*)
Cecropin-4	[103]	GWLKKIGKKIERVGQNTRDATIQ AIGVAQQAANVAATLKG (40aa)	AH	4	*4*	Synthetic peptide
Myxinidin 2	[104]	KIKWILKYWKWS (12aa)	AH	—	*12.5*	*Myxine glutinosa L*
Myxinidin 3		RIRWILRYWRWS (12aa)	B-sheet	—	*6.3*	
FLIP 7	[105]	???				*Calliphora vicina* (Medicinal Maggots)
Mastoparan	[65, 106, 107]	INLKALAALAKKIL (14aa)	AH	4	—	*Vespula lewisii* (Hornet venom)

Peptide	Ref.	Sequence	Structure	MIC against *A. baumannii* (μg/mL)		Source
				Antibiotic-susceptible	MDR	
Mastoparan-AF (EMP-AF)	[108]	INLKAIAALAKKLF-NH2 (14aa)	AH	2–16	2–16	Hornet venom (*Vespa affinis*)
Histatin-8	[65]	KFHEKHHSHRGY (12aa)	AH	8	—	*H. sapiens*
DCD-1 L	[109, 110]	SSLLEKGLDGAKKAVGGLGKLGK DAVEDLESVGKGAVHDVKDVLD SVL (48aa)	AH	16	—	Eccrine sweat glands
Tachyplesin III	[84]	KWCFRVCYRGICYRKCR-NH2 (17aa)	B-sheet 2 dissulfite bridges	—	—	Horseshoe crabs (*Tachypleus gigas*) and (*Carcinoscorpius rotundicauda*)
RR	[111, 112]	WLRRIKAWLRR (11aa)	AH	—	25–99	Computationally designed
RR2	[112]	WIRRIKKWIRRVHK (14aa)	AH	—	3–6	
RR-4	[112]	WLRRIKAWLRRIKA (14aa)	Ah	—	3–6	
DP7	[113–115]		AH	—	4–16	
Omega 76-shuft1	[116]	AFLLKKKKGIIFFEKAKKGK	AH	—	4–16	
'Ω17 family peptides	[116]	RKKAIKLVKKLVKKLKKALK(20aa)	AH	2	1–8	
'Ω76 family peptides	[116]	FLKAIKKFGKEFKKIGAKLK (20aa)	AH	4	2–8	
Stapled AMP Mag (i + 4)1, 15(A9 K, B21A, N22 K, S23 K)	[117]	Mag(i + 4)1,15(A9K,B21A,N22K,S23K)	complex	—	—	NA, based in magainin 2 structure

Peptide	Ref.	Sequence	Structure	MIC against *A. baumannii* (μg/mL)		Source
				Antibiotic-susceptible	MDR	
PNA (RXR)4 XB	[118]	—	—	—	—	Peptide nucleic acid conjugated to (RXR)4 Phosphorodiamidate Morpholino Oligomers
HP(2–9)-ME(1–12) (HPME)	[119]	AKKVFKRLGIGAVLKVLTTG (20aa)	AH	6.25	3.12–12.5	Chimeric peptide
HP(2–9)-MA(1–12) (HPMA)		AKKVFKRLGIGKFLHSAKKF-NH_2 (20aa)	AH	6.25	3.12–6.25	Chimeric peptide
CA(1–8)-ME(1–12) (CAME)		KWKLFKKIGIGAVLKVLTTG-NH_2 (20aa)	Ah	3.12	3.12–12.5	Chimeric peptide
CA(1–8)-MA(1–12) (CAMA)		KWKLFKKIGIGKFLHSAKKF-NH_2 (20aa)	AH	12.5	3.12–12.5	Chimeric peptide
Hp 1404 analogs (A, K, V, L, I, W)	[120, 121]	GILGKLWEGVKSIF-NH_2 (14aa)	AH	3.13–12.5	3.13–16.25	Venom gland scorpion (*Heterometnus pertersii)*
Octominin	[122]	GWLIRGAIHAGKAIHGLIHRRRH (23aa)	AH	—	5	Synthetic derived, defensin 3 of *Octopus minor*
Ceragenins; CSA-192; CSA-131; D-150-177C; HBcARDderivative	[123]	Steroids compounds	???	—	—	Cholic acid synthetic mimics,
Protegrin-1	[124]	RGGRLCYCRRRFCVCVGR-NH2(18aa)	AH	—	—	*Cimex lectularius*
S4A	[125]	IOWAGOLFOLFO-NH2	AH	100	50	NA
SPO		NINONWNANGNONLNFNONLNF NO-NH2		100	50	

Peptide	Ref.	Sequence	Structure	MIC against *A. baumannii* (μg/mL)		Source
				Antibiotic-susceptible	MDR	
Nuripep 1653	[126]	VRGLAPKKSLWPFGGPFKSPFN (22aa)	AH	—	12	Derived from the P54 nutrient reservoir protein (aa 271–292) pea protein from *Pisum sativum*
Agelaia-MPI	[127]	INWLKLGKAIIDAL (14aa)	AH	6.25	12.5–25	*Agelaia pallipes pallipes*
Polybia-MPII	[127]	INWLKLGKMVIDAL (14aa)	AH	12.5	25	*Pseudopolybia vespiceps testacea*
Polydin-I	[127]	AVAGEKLWLLPHLLKMLLTPTP (22aa)	AH	>25	>25	*Polybia dimorpha* (*Social wasp*)
Con10	[127]	FWSFLVKAASKILPSLIGGGDDNK SSS (27aa)	AH	12.5	12.5	Scorpion venoms (*Opisthacanthus cayaporum*)
NDBP5.8		GILGKIWEGVKSLI (14aa)		>25	>25	
Delfibactin A	[128]	$C_{40}H_{68}N_{14}O_{18}$	—	—	16	Gram-negative bactéria *Delfia* spp.
WLBU2- arginine-rich amphiphilic peptide	[129]	RRWVRRVRRWVRRVVRVVRRWV RR (24aa)	—	~7.484	~7.484	Skin wounds
α-Helical-26 (A12L/A20L)	[130]	Ac-KWKSFLKTFKSLKKTVLHTLLK AISS-NH2	AH	—	0.5–1.0	D- and L-diastereomeric peptides
Cy02 (cyclotide)	[131]	???	???	???	???	*Viola odorata*
Bicarinalin (YRTX-Tb1a)	[132]	KiKIPWGKVKDFLVGGMKAV (20aa)	AH	—	4	*Tetramorium bicarinatum* venom
BP100		KKLFKKILKYL (11aa)	AH	—	4	

Peptide	Ref.	Sequence	Structure	MIC against *A. baumannii* (μg/mL)		Source
				Antibiotic-susceptible	**MDR**	
Glatiramer acetate (synthetic COP-1)	[132]	synthetic	—	Reduct viable cells	Reduct viable cells	*Homo sapiens*
Lactoperoxidase (Lpo)	[133]	Large protein	complex	—	Inhibition effects, significant clearance of *A. baumannii* in lung and blood culture	Camel (Colostrum milk)
Lactoferrin (Lf)		Large protein	complex	—		
Artlysin Art-175	[134]	Comprises a modified variant of endolysin KZ144 with an N-terminal fusion to SMAP-29		—	4–20	*Pseudomonas aeruginosa* bacteriophage
Epsilon-poly L-lysine (EPL)-catechol	[135]	Complex	???	—	Reducing bacterial burden *in vivo*	*Streptomyces albulus* derived
Chex1-Arg20 amide (ARV-1502)	[136]	H-Chex-Arg-Pro-Asp-Lys-Pro-Arg-Pro-Tyr-Leu-Pro-Arg-Pro-Arg-Pro-Pro-ArgPro-Val-Arg-NH2	???	—	Reduction of bacterial load	NA
I16K-piscidin-1 and analogs	[137]	FFHHIFRGIVHVGKTIHRLVTG (22aa)	???	—	3.1	Hybrid striped bass *Morone saxatilis x M. chrysops*
Nodule-specific cysteine-rich (NCR) peptide and its derivatives	[138]	RNGCIVDPRCPYQQCRRPLYCRRR (24aa)	AH	1.6–25 MBC	—	*Medicago trunculata*
TAT-RasGAP$_{317-326}$ anticancer peptide	[139]	G48RKKRRQRRR^{57} + W^{317}MWVTNLRTD^{326}	AH	Growth inhibitory effect	—	Chimeric (cell penetrating sequence + Src homology sequence)

Peptide	Ref.	Sequence	Structure	MIC against *A. baumannii* (µg/mL)		Source
				Antibiotic-susceptible	**MDR**	
D-150-177C, HBcARD derivative peptide	[140]	RRRGRSPRRRTPSPRRRRSQSPRR RRSC (28AA)	AH	16	16–32	*Hepatitis B* virus
Colistin (Polymyxin E)	[141]	C52H98N16O13 (cyclic compound)	≠	Antibiofilm, side effects		*Bacillus colistinus*
PlyF307 (P307)	[142]	146 aa (Access number KJ740396)	?	750	750–2000	*Phage Lysin*
P307^{SQ-8C}		NAKDYKGAAAEFPKWNKAGGRV LAGLVKRRKSQSRESQC (39aa)	???	125	62.5–125	Hepatitis B virus
N10	[143]	ACKDVNTSMCGGK (13aa)	AH	500	500	Blood biopanning
NB2		ACERSIRTVCGGK (13aa)	AH	500	500	Biofilm biopanning
Melittin with imipenem (IPM)	[144]	GIGAVLKVLTTGLPALISWIKRKR QQ (26aa) + IPM	AH	0.31–0.37	0.12–0.25	European honeybee and antimicrobial
Melittin with colistin (COL)		GIGAVLKVLTTGLPALISWIKRKR QQ (26aa) + COL	AH	0.37–0.5	0.19–0.37	

NA, not available; AH, alpha helical; IPM, imipenem; COL, colistin.

Table 1.
*List of AMP with activity anti-*A. baumannii.

an *ex vivo* human skin infection model and an *in vivo* murine skin infection model at concentrations above 5% [74].

2.1.2 Snake cathelicidins

The anti-*A. baumannii* activity among the cathelicidins isolated from snakes has been reported for the peptides cathelicidin-BF (Cath-BF) [75] and *Naja atra* cathelicidin (NA-CATH). One of the best-known cathelicidins is Cath-BF having an α-helical structure, isolated from the venous glands of the species *Bungatus fasciatus* [152]. It has been shown that Cath-BF causes bacterial death through two bacterial membrane disruption mechanisms and attacking intracellular targets [152]. According to available reports, this peptide is highly active against drug-resistant clinical isolates of *A. baumannii*, inhibiting its growth around 12.8 μg/ml concentration [75]. ZY4 cathelicidin-BF-15 derived, a cyclic peptide stabilized by a disulfide bridge with high stability *in vivo* (the half-life is 1.8 h), showed excellent activity against *A. baumannii*, including standard clinical MDR strains with MIC values ranging between 4.6 and 9.4 μg/mL. ZY4 killed bacteria by permeabilizing the bacterial membrane showed a low propensity to induce resistance, exhibited biofilm inhibition and eradication activities, and killed persister cells [76]. The peptide NA-CATH, produced by a cobra called *N. atra*, possesses an α-helical structure at N-terminal and an unstructured segment at C-terminal [77, 153]. This peptide exerts antimicrobial activity through the membrane lysis by membrane thinning or transient pore formation [154] and is highly active against drug-resistant and sensitive *A. baumannii* strains, completely inhibiting bacterial growth at a concentration of 10 μg/ml [77, 153]. In 2018, Zhao et al. identified a novel cathelicidin (OH-CATH) from the king cobra, with its analog DOH-CATH30 found to exhibit potent microbicidal activity (MIC 1.56 to 12.5 μg/mL) against several Gram-negative and Gram-positive bacteria, including MDR *A. baumannii* [78]. Other cathelicidins with antimicrobial activity, identified in the venous glands, are OH-CATH30, from the venom of the cobra and mirtoxin, from *Myrmecia pilosula* [78, 79], presenting antimicrobial activity through inhibition of planktonic bacterial growth and biofilm, eradication of persistent bacterial cells, and inhibition of inflammatory process [76, 78].

Compounds with similar activity have been identified in the venom of some scorpion species and tested against antibiotic-resistant bacteria. Therefore, Al-Asmari et al. evaluate the *in vitro* antimicrobial activities of the toxins extracted from three medically necessary Saudi Scorpions. Among these, only *Leiurus quinquestriatus* showed significant broad-spectrum antimicrobial activity in a dose-dependent manner from 5 to 20 mg/mL, inhibiting 50.6% of growth and survival of MDR *A. baumannii* [80]. High antimicrobial activity was also observed for AMPs ranalexin and danalexin obtained from *Rana catesbeiana* [81], LS-sarcotoxin, and LS-stomoxyn (*Lucilla serricata*) [82], and minibactenecins *(Capra hircus)* [83]. However, further *in vivo* studies are needed to improve the pharmacokinetics of systemic administration and find solutions to avoid their degradation by proteases despite the antimicrobial activity on *A. baumannii* strains of these compounds.

2.1.3 Alligator cathelicidins

Alligator mississippiensis (American alligator), a member of order Crocodilia, lives in bacteria-laden environments but cannot often succumb to bacterial infections. Serum of alligators has antibacterial activity beyond that of human sérum [155], killing a wide range of pathogens, and it is believed that this activity is attributable at least partially to the presence of CAMPs in the alligator plasma and extracts [156]. A study by Barksdale et al. (2017) reported the anti-*A. baumannii* effect of AMPs produced by American alligator: cathelicidin called AM-CATH36 and its two fragments including AM-CATH28 and AM-CATH21 [77]. Alligator cathelicidin can inhibit the growth of both drug-resistant and sensitive *A. baumannii* at the 2.5 μg/ml concentration. Furthermore, two shorter fragments of this peptide can inhibit the drug-resistant *A. baumannii* at a 10 μg/ml concentration. The anti-*A. baumannii* effect of these three peptides is through membrane permeabilization. Interestingly, MDR clinical isolates of *A. baumannii* were more susceptible to both the AM CATH21 and AM-CATH28 peptides than the sensitive strains.

2.1.4 Wallaby antimicrobial

The marsupial AMP Wallaby antimicrobial 1 (WAM-1) is a cathelicidin isolated from the mammary gland of the Tammar wallaby (*Macropus eugenii*) with antibacterial and antifungal activities with high potential to combat drug-resistant pathogens [84, 157]. Spencer et al. (2018) studied the AMP LL-37 and WARM-1 effects on MDR *A. baumannii*, and both peptides were able to inhibit biofilm formation in all clinical isolates at some concentrations of WAM-1 effectively dispersed 24-h biofilms in most isolates tested, including MDR strains [85]. The antibacterial effects of LL-37are diminished in the presence of human serum. However, this is not the case with WAM-1. Although the mechanism of action has yet to be determined, WAM-1 has been shown *in vitro* to be 12 to 80 times more effective than LL-37 in its ability to kill several bacterial pathogens, including several clinical isolates of *A. baumannii*. Unlike LL-37, WAM-1 is not inhibited by high NaCl concentrations and does not cause hemolysis in human red blood cells (RBC), so it has the potential to be used for *in vivo* applications [85].

2.1.5 Bovine cathelicidins (Indolicidin and Bactenecin)

Indolicidin is a short tryptophan-rich cationic AMP encoded by a member of the cathelicidin gene family, isolated from cytoplasmic granules of the bovine neutrophils [158, 159]. Indolicidin acts by displacing divalent cations from their binding sites on the surface of the cell membrane and causes bacterial death through channel formation in the cytoplasmic membrane [88]. Indolicidin not only forms pores in the membrane but can also inhibit DNA processing enzymes [160, 161]. This peptide is among the potent anti-*A. baumannii* AMPs with MIC of 4–32 and 16 μg/ml against sensitive and colistin-resistant clinical isolates, respectively [86]. In a study by Giacometti et al. were investigated the *in vitro* activity of indolicidin and other AMPs alone and in combination with antimicrobial agents, the MIC of indolicidin against 12 MDR clinical isolates was reported as 2–64 μg/ml [87]. Isolated from bovine, ovine, and caprine neutrophil granules, Bactenecin is a short cyclic, arginine-rich cationic AMP [89] with a type I β-turn structure and forms a loop due to the disulfide bond between cysteines 3 and 11 [90]. These AMPs act by permeabilizing the cell membrane and inhibiting protein and RNA synthesis in bacteria [70]. Vila-Farres et al. (2012) reported the anti-*A. baumannii* effect of this peptide can inhibit sensitive and colistin-resistant strains of *A. baumannii* at 16 and 64 μg/ml, respectively [86].

2.2 Defensins

Defensins are an evolutionarily ancient class of AMPs present in animals, plants, and fungi involved in the immune system of living organisms and contain six (invertebrates) to eight conserved cysteine residues in their structure. They are categorized into three subfamilies of α, β, and θ-defensins [162]. Most defensins bind to the cell membrane and make pores, leading to bacterial death [163].

2.2.1 α-Defensins (HNPs and HD5)

The subfamily of human neutrophil peptides (HNPs), also known as α-defensins, are secreted and released from polymorphonuclear neutrophil (PMN) granules upon activation and are conventionally involved in microbial killing [164]. Two important CAMPs HNP-1 and HNP-2, which differ in only one initial amino acid, can inhibit the growth of the standard strain of *A. baumannii* ATCC 19606 at a concentration of 50 μg/ml. Interestingly, the colistin-resistant mutant of *A. baumannii* ATCC 19606 is much more sensitive (MIC = 3.25 μg/ml) to HNP-1 than the standard strain [86]. Human defensin 5 (HD5) has a relatively low anti-*A. baumannii* effect (MIC = 320 μg/ml). However, an analog called HD5d5 obtained by sequence modification presented a stronger bactericidal effect (MIC = 40 μg / ml) against *A. baumannii*, exerting the effect through damage to the membrane, accumulation in the cytoplasm, and reduction of catalase and superoxide dismutase activities [165, 166].

2.2.2 β-Defensins

Human β-Defensin (HBD) 2, 3 of this subfamily have anti-*Acinetobacter* effects. HBD-2 is primarily produced by the epithelial lining of the respiratory and urinary tracts, and engaging is more effective on MDR clinical isolates than non-MDR isolates [167]. Longer than most of the natural AMPs, HBD-3 combined helix and β structure [147]. Even though the anti-*Acinetobacter* bactericidal effect is inhibited by exposure to human serum, it can kill all MDR and non-MDR *A. baumannii* clinical isolates at 4 μg/ml during 1.5 h in the serum-free environment. Thus, this peptide has the potential to be further studied for wounds infected by *A. baumannii* since it demonstrated wound-healing effects [97, 168].

2.2.3 α-Helical and antiparallel β-sheet defensins

CL-defensin, belonging to the family of insect defensins, is predicted to have a characteristic N-terminal loop, an α-helix, and an antiparallel β-sheet, which was supported by circular dichroism spectroscopy [95]. In addition, this peptide induces pore formation in other Gram-positive bacteria and causes a small amount of membrane permeabilization in *A. baumannii* [95].

2.3 Frog antimicrobial peptides

2.3.1 Magainin and pexiganan (its analog)

The Magainin-1 and 2 are cationic, α-helical, and amphipathic AMPs ionophores isolated from the skin of the African clawed frog (*Xenopus laevis*) [168, 169]. The primary mechanism of antimicrobial activity is probably pore formation in outer and inner membranes, although the exact mechanism of action is not yet precise [98, 170]. Despite both have anti-*Acinetobacter* training, Magainin-2 is much stronger and able to inhibit the growth of sensitive and MDR strains of *A. baumannii* at 4.9–64 μg/ml, while reported as 256 μg/ml for Magainin-1 [86, 98]. Magainin-2 has some advantages, such as anticancer effect, stability at physiological salt concentrations, lack of hemolytic activity, and toxicity for mammalian cells [98]. Furthermore, Magainin-2 can inhibit and eliminate the biofilm of *A. baumannii* [98]. Pexiganan AMP or MSI-78 is a synthetic analog of Magainin-2 with a potent and broad spectrum of action [171, 172]; it kills bacteria by forming toroidal pores in their cell membranes [172, 173]. Several studies have been performed on anti-*Acinetobacter* activity due to its being highly active against *Acinetobacter*. Pexiganan can inhibit the growth of MDR and sensitive clinical isolates of A. *baumannii* at a concentration of 1–8 μg/ml [100, 101, 174]. Jáskiewicz et al. studied the antimicrobial activity of eight peptides on *A. baumannii* ATCC 19606 reference strains. Among these, CAMEL and pexiganan showed potent antimicrobial and anti-biofilm activity [102].

2.3.2 Brevinin-2 related peptide (B2RP)

B2RP is an α-helical AMP isolated from the skin secretions of the mink frog *Rana septentrionalis* [175] and carpenter frog Rana virgatipes [176]. This peptide forms an α-helical structure adjacent to the target cell, resulting in the perturbation of the phospholipid bilayer that may lead to growth inhibition of bacterial death, and the application of this peptide for systemic use is limited due to the moderate toxicity for human red blood cells [177]. B2RP inhibited the growth of a susceptible strain of *A. baumannii* at 29 μg/ml concentration but inhibited the MDR isolates more efficiently at 7–13.9 μg/ml [103]. The analogs of these peptides (D4K, K16A, L18K) resulted in twofolds higher anti-*A. baumannii* activity and much lower hemolytic activity [103]. A study reported that the analog of B2RP with D4K substitution inhibited sensitive and colistin-resistant [103] and XDR isolates of *A. baumannii* [105].

2.3.3 B2RP-ERa

B2RP-ERa is a cationic AMP from the Brevinin family isolated from the skin of the Asian frog *Hylarana erythraea* [106, 178]. Shorter and with lower molecular weight, B2RP-ERa is structurally similar to B2RP. B2RP-ERa is an anti-inflammatory peptide with no toxic effect on peripheral blood mononuclear cells [179] with low hemolytic activity [178], which could inhibit the growth of sensitive and drug-resistant *Acinetobacter* strains at 8–32 and 8–64 μg/ml, respectively [104, 106].

2.3.4 Alyteserins

Alyteserins are a class of cationic AMPs, which firstly reported their presence in norepinephrine-stimulated skin secretions of the midwife toad [180]. However, initial studies show that Alyteserin-1c has more significant inhibitory activity against Gram-negative bacteria, while Alyteserin-2a is more active against Gram-positive bacteria [180], the anti-*A. baumannii* effects of these Alyteserins have already been proven [107, 108]. Alyteserin-1c is a cationic α-helical AMP with low hemolytic activity on human red blood cells firstly isolated from *Alytes obstetricans* [107, 180, 181]. The MIC and MBC against clinical isolates of MDR *A. baumannii* have been reported as 11.3–22.6 μg/ml [107]. Substitution of E4K on this AMP reduced the hemolytic activity, and enhanced the antimicrobial and cationic activity [107]. The analog [E4K] inhibits the growth of colistin-sensitive, colistin-resistant, and XDR *A. baumannii* isolates at concentrations of 4–16 μg/ml, 4–16 μg/ml [104], and 8–64 μg/ml, respectively [105]. Alyteserin-2a is also a tiny α-helical AMP that displays relatively weak antimicrobial and hemolytic activities. Despite its anti-*A. baumannii* potential was not high mainly, some structural changes resulted in lower toxicity against human erythrocytes and higher bactericidal effect (4–8 folds) against MDR isolates with MIC of 6.8–13.6 μg/ml [108].

2.3.5 Peptide glycine-leucine-amide

AM1 (PGLa-AM1) PGLa-AM1 is another Anti-*Acinetobacter* AMP isolated from the frog *Xenopus amieti*. In addition to the low hemolytic activity, it is also active against other pathogens, including *E. coli* and *S. aureus* [104, 106, 109], and can kill sensitive and colistin-resistant *A. baumannii* isolates at 16–128 μg/ ml concentration [104].

2.3.6 Caerulein precursor fragment (CPF)

CPF-AM1 is a cationic AMP firstly isolated from *X. amieti* [110]. This peptide is capable of bacterial binding LPS and has activity against Gram-negative and Gram-positive bacteria, primarily oral and respiratory pathogens, with advantages such as low hemolytic activity and lack of toxicity against fibroblast cells [109]. This anti-*A. baumannii* peptide inhibits the growth of sensitive and colistin-resistant strains at 16–128 and 4–128 μg/ml, respectively [104, 114]. CPF-B1, isolated from Marsabit clawed frog *Xenopus borealis*, is another anti-*A. baumannii* member of this family with low hemolytic activity. This peptide inhibits MDR *A. baumannii* clinical isolates at concentrations of 11.4–22.8 μg/ml [112]. Finally, CPF-C1 is a peptide member of this family with proved anti-*A. baumannii* effect with inhibitory activity against the strain at 5 μg/ml concentration [111].

2.3.7 Hymenochirins

Hymenochirins are a class of AMPs produced by two frogs of *Pseudhymenochirus merlini* and *Hymenochirus boettgeri* with letters P and B in the second part name of these peptides indicating the producing species of the peptide, respectively [37, 182]. Hymenochirin-1B is a cationic, α-helical amphibian host-defense peptide with antimicrobial, anticancer, and immunomodulatory properties. This peptide has anti-*A. baumannii* properties against MDR isolates with MIC of 19.1 μg/ml [113]. Among the analogs of hymenochirin-1B obtained by amino acid substitution method, [E6k and D9k] hymenochirin-1B reduced human erythrocytes' toxicity and showed 3.9-folds higher activity against *A. baumannii.* [E6k and D9k] hymenochirin-1B is active against both MDR and XDR isolates and could inhibit the growth of these isolates at 4.9 μg/ml concentration [113]. Hymenochirin-1 Pa is another cationic member of this family with moderate hemolytic activity. This peptide inhibited the growth of XDR *A. baumannii* isolates at 7.5–15 μg/ml concentration [114, 182].

2.3.8 XT-7

XT-7 was first isolated from norepinephrine-stimulated skin secretions of *Xenopus tropicalis* [183]. The activity anti-*Acinetobacte*of this peptide was first reported against A. baumannii Euroclone I NM8 strain (MIC = 22.2 μg/ml) [111]. Later, the amino acid substitution of lysine at position 4 [G4K] increased the therapeutic index [115] principally. Subsequent studies were based on this new analog that inhibited sensitive and drug-resistant *A. baumannii* strains at concentrations of 4–32 and 4–64 μg/ml, respectively [104].

2.3.9 Buforins

Buforin II is a potent antimicrobial peptide derived from Burforin I, isolated from the stomach tissue of the Asian toad *Bufo gargarizans* [184]. It causes bacterial death by crossing the membrane, binding to intracellular targets, including DNA and RNA, and inhibiting cellular functions [116]. This peptide has a potent anti-*Acinetobacter* activity since it can hinder the growth of both sensitive and resistant isolates of *A. baumannii* at concentrations of 0.25–39 μg/ml [87, 98]. Buforin II alone or in combination with an antibiotic showed highly potent on *A. baumannii* sepsis treatment in a rat model [104].

2.4 Melittin

Melittin is a cationic amphipathic α-helical AMP isolated from the venom (approximately 50% of the dry weight) of the European honeybee (*Apis mellifera*) [185] with numerous reported properties such as antifungal [186], antiparasitic [187], antibacterial [185], antiviral, and anticancer properties [188]. The primary mechanism of melittin action is the membrane lysis through pore formation (a carpet-like mechanism) [189]. This potent anti-*Acinetobacter* peptide inhibits MDR and XDR clinical isolates at 0.125–2 μg/ml concentration [118, 119]. A study demonstrated that topical administration of melittin at concentrations of 16 and 32 μg/mL in mice killed 93.3% and 100% of an XDR *A. baumannii* on a third-degree burned area, respectively [118]. No toxicity was observed on the injured or healthy derma and circulating red blood cells in the examined mice. Recently, a study that evaluated the melittin against Brazilian clinical strains revealed that most strains were susceptible, except for one pan drug-resistant strain [190].

2.5 Cecropins

Cecropins, the lytic peptides, were initially isolated from the hemolymph of the giant silk moth, *Hyalophora cecropia*, and possess antibacterial and anticancer activity *in vitro* [191, 192]. The primary antimicrobial mechanism of cecropins is membrane lysis [193]. Cecropin A is a cationic amphipathic α-helical AMP that can induce apoptosis by oxidative stress in addition to attacking the membrane [194]. This peptide has potent antimicrobial activity against *A. baumannii*, inhibiting MDR clinical isolates at 0.5–32 μg/ml [99]. Vila-Farres et al. reported that this peptide inhibited the growth of sensitive and colistin-resistant strains of *A. baumannii* at 32 and 256 μg/ ml, respectively [86]. A pilot study that evaluated the viability of *Caenorhabditis elegans* infected by *A. baumannii* in the presence of 68 insect-derived AMPs identified 15 cecropin or cecropin-like peptides that prolonged the survival of worms infected with *A. baumannii* [121]. Interestingly, the direct investigation of the anti-*Acinetobacter* effect also showed that these 15 AMPs could inhibit the growth of *A. baumannii* at 4.5 to over 20 μg/ml concentrations. BR003-cecropin A, isolated from *Aedes aegypti*, is the most active member of this group. This peptide inhibited sensitive and MDR *A. baumannii* strains at 4.5 μg/ml [100]. Musca domestica cecropin (Mdc) isolated from the *larvae* of a housefly inhibits both standard (ATCC 19606) and MDR strains of *A. baumannii* at 4 μg/ml with high speed (half an hour) [122]. Cecropin P1, an AMP isolated from *Ascaris suum* of pig intestine, showed high activity against colistin-sensitive *A. baumannii* with MIC at 1.6 μg/ml. In contrast, there was less activity against the colistin-resistant strains with MIC >25 μg/ml [86].

Other peptides that showed great activity against susceptible MDR and extensively drug-resistant (XDR) *A. baumannii* strains were Cecropin-4, an α-helical synthetic AMP [124], and CAMEL, a hybrid AMP consisting of cecropin from *H. cecropia* and melittin from *Apis melífera* [102]. In addition, AMPs with activity against biofilms have been observed in cecropins identified in *M. domestica* [124], myxinidin isolated from *Myxine glutinosa* [104], and in the naturally occurring AMP complex isolated from the maggots of blowfly *Calliphora vicina* (Diptera, *Calliphoridae*) named FLIP7 (Fly Larvae Immune Peptides 7) [126].

2.6 Mastoparan

Mastoparan is a small cationic amphipathic α-helical AMP isolated from the hornet venom of *Vespula lewisii* [195, 196] with a robust anti-*Acinetobacter* activity. However, the anti-*acinetobacter* solid activity, the high hemolytic activity, and toxic effects affected highly therapeutic applications [197]. Mastoparan inhibited the growth of a sensitive wild-type *A. baumannii* ATCC 19606 and a colistin-resistant *A. baumannii* ATCC 19606 mutant at 4 and 1 μg/ml, respectively. This study also used 14 colistin-susceptible *A. baumannii* clinical isolates and 13 pan-resistant *A. baumannii* strains isolated in a hospital outbreak [198] and reported the MIC of 1–16 and 2–8 μg/ ml for sensitive and colistin-resistant isolates, respectively [86]. Mastoparan-AF (MP-AF), isolated from the hornet venom of *Vespa affinis*, also showed effective antimicrobial activity with MICs ranging from 2 to 16 μg/ml against MDR *A. baumannii* isolates [129]. Analogs of mastoparan were made to increase the stability of the peptide in serum. These analogs had an equal inhibitory effect with mastoparan against XDR *A. baumannii* strains (4 μg/ml); in addition, it showed stability in the presence of human serum for more than 24 h [86].

2.7 Histatins

Histatins belong to a distinct family of at least 12 low-molecular weight, histidine-rich cationic, salivary gland peptides with antimicrobial effect through the plasma membrane disruption [199]. Histatin-8, known as hemagglutination-inhibiting peptide [200], was the only member of this group that showed antimicrobial activity against *A. baumannii*, inhibiting the growth of both sensitive standard strains colistin-resistant mutant *A. baumannii* ATCC 19606 at 32 μg/ml [86].

2.8 Dermcidins

Dermcidin is an anionic AMP encoded by the DCD gene in humans essentially produced in eccrine sweat glands, secreted into a sweat, and further transported to the skin's epidermal surface [130, 201]. It has two parts; N-terminal peptide promotes neural cell survival under severe oxidative stress conditions called DCD-1 L [130]. DCD-1 L, a C-terminal peptide with the net electric charge of −2, is the only anionic anti-*Acinetobacter* natural AMP found in the literature that shows partial helicity in solution [130, 182]. Interestingly, in exposure to this AMP, the PDR *A. baumannii* isolates are twice more susceptible as XDR isolates and the standard strain (ATCC 19606) (MIC = 8 μg/ ml) [131].

2.9 Tachyplesin III

Tachyplesin III, isolated from the hemolymph of the Southeast Asian horseshoe crabs *Tachypleus gigas* and *Carcinoscorpius rotundicauda*, consists of 17 amino acids with two disulfide bridges and is a representative antimicrobial peptide with a cyclic β-sheet structure. However, its potential toxicity hampers its use in mammalian cells [202]. Nevertheless, Tachyplesin III could inhibit the

XDR *A. baumannii* strains (8–16 μg/ml) and at 2 × MIC, eliminating the XDR *A. baumannii* strains [203].

2.10 Computationally designed antimicrobial peptide

The biosynthesis of AMPs can be a starting point for obtaining AMPS with functions similar to natural ones, being an attractive therapeutic option for preventing and controlling infections. In this sense, bioinformatics and computer science have been widely used in various aspects in many studies of *A. baumannii*, such as design evaluation of AMPs [136, 204–208], which includes two general principles that increased antimicrobial activity and reduced toxicity against eukaryotic cells [209, 210]. As an example of synthetic AMPs, we have stapled AMP [137] and PNA (RXR) 4XB, an antisense nucleic acid peptide compound [138] with intense bactericidal activity. The synthetic RR is a small α-helical AMP with fast bactericidal activity capable of retaining the antimicrobial property at physiological concentrations of NaCl and MgCl2 [132]. The anti-*A. baumannii* effect of RR against sensitive and MDR strains inhibits the growth at 25–99 μg/ml concentration. Two new analogs of this peptide were introduced with much stronger anti-*A. baumannii* properties than RR, and the AMPs RR2 and RR4 inhibit the growth of sensitive and drug-resistant strains (3–6 μg/ml) [211]. The peptide DP7 inhibits the growth of antibiotic-resistant *A. baumannii* strains at 4–16 μg/ml concentration, and the synergistic effects were showed after simultaneous treatment of some drug-resistant *A. baumannii* isolates with DP7 and antibiotics such as amoxicillin, azithromycin, and vancomycin [133]. Zhang et al. showed that DP7 invades the microbial cell through various pathways after sequencing the transcriptome of the bacteria exposed to this peptide [134]. Omega76 is a cationic AMP with an α-helical structure, causing death in *A. baumannii* through membrane disruption. This peptide was designed based on the maximum common subgraph of helices and further introduced as an appropriate alternative for colistin due to its high anti-*A. baumannii* activity against carbapenem and tigecycline-resistant isolates (MBC = 2–8 μg/ml) and lack of toxicity in the mouse model [135].

3. Resistance to AMPS

Although AMPs have a low likelihood to select for resistance, similar to the conventional antibiotics, another challenge is represented by the numerous reports describing the development of resistance mechanisms against some AMPs, including proteolytic degradation or sequestration by secreted proteins, impedance by exopolymers, and biofilm matrix molecules, circumvention of attraction by cell surface/membrane alteration, and export by efflux pumps [212–216]. The development of resistance to colistin by *A. baumannii* following long-term clinical application was observed [217, 218]. In *A. baumannii* stable colistin resistance was also observed following direct plating with the complete loss of LPS production due to the inactivation of one of three genes involved in lipid A biosynthesis (*lpxA, lpxD, or lpxC*). Resistance to colistin is an important clinical issue, considering that colistin is a last-resort drug used to treat MDR nosocomial pathogens [218–220]. Several mechanisms have been reported responsible for resistance to AMPs, including expression of efflux pumps, increased secretion of proteolytic enzymes, and surface charge modification to avoid membrane-peptide electrostatic interactions [213, 221, 222].

For delivering the AMPs, several nanocarriers were developed, which may help avoid the low bioavailability, proteolysis, or susceptibility and toxicity associated with APMs [223, 224]. Changes in the molecular structure, modifications of biochemical characterization, and combination with common antibiotics have been reported to reduce AMP resistance [214]. The aprotinin is the first inhibitor identified to inhibit AMP resistance in multiple pathogens [225].

4. Conclusion(s)

A. baumannii is one of the ESKCAPE pathogens responsible for nosocomial and community-acquired infections, with the incidence of MDR and virulent clones increasingly worldwide. The enormous adaptability of *A. baumannii*, as well as the remarkable ability to acquire determinants of resistance, allied to your innate ability to form biofilms, contributes to the inefficiency of most current therapeutic strategies, determining the transition to the "post-antibiotic era" and highlighting the necessity to develop new therapeutic approaches. In this context, natural and synthetic AMPs emerge as potential next-generation antibiotics to mitigate a wide array of microbial infections, including those caused by MDR *A. baumannii* strains. Moreover, the antimicrobial activity of these peptides can be effectively increased by minor modifications through the development of computer science and bioinformatics. The synthetic AMPs present a promising solution to overcome the drawbacks of using natural AMPs. They contain critical features based on natural AMPs, with slight modifications to achieve higher antimicrobial efficiency and improved chemical stability. In this research, we observed the main properties of anti-*A. baumannii* peptides with some common characteristics, such as 1. The α-helical structure was predominant. 2. Most peptides have a positive charge, and in many cases, there is a direct relationship between an increased positive charge and your activity. 3. The action mechanisms of these peptides are direct membrane attack and intracellular targeting or both simultaneously. Unfortunately, considerable experimental data describe how bacteria can develop resistance to AMPs, such as colistin and polymyxin B in *A. baumannii*. Since AMPS are considered potential novel antimicrobial drugs, understanding the mechanism of bacterial resistance to direct killing of AMPS is of great significance.

Conflict of interest

The authors declare no conflict of interest.

Notes/thanks/other declarations

We thank D. Guilherme Curty Lechuga by the drawing of figures 1 and 2 of this chapter.

DOI: http://dx.doi.org/10.5772/intechopen.100389

Author details

Karyne Rangel[1] and Salvatore Giovanni De-Simone[1,2,3*]

1 Center for Technological Development in Health (CDTS)/National Institute of Science and Technology for Innovation in Neglected Diseases Populations (INCT-IDPN), FIOCRUZ, Rio de Janeiro, Brazil

2 Epidemiology and Molecular Systematics Laboratory, Oswaldo Cruz Institute, FIOCRUZ, Rio de Janeiro, Brazil

3 Biology Institute, Molecular and Cellular Biology, Department, Federal Fluminense University, Niterói, Brazil

*Address all correspondence to: dsimone@cdts.fiocruz.br

References

[1] O'Neill J. Tackling Drug-Resistance Infections Globally: Final Report and Recommendations. The Review on Antimicrobial Resistance. London, UK: Government of the United Kingdom; 2016. 84 p

[2] Tacconelli E, Carrara A, Savoldi S, Harbarth M, Mendelson DL, Monnet C, et al. Discovery, research, and development of new antibiotics: The WHO priority list of antibiotic-resistant bacteria and tuberculosis. The Lancet Infectious Diseases. 2018;**18**(3):318-327

[3] Lewis K. Persister cells, dormancy, and infectious disease. Nature Reviews. Microbiology. 2007;**5**(1):48-56

[4] Lewis K. Persister cells. Annual Review of Microbiology. 2010;**64**:357-372. DOI: 10.1146/annurev.micro.112408.134306

[5] Fernández L, Breidenstein EBM, Hancock REW. Importance of adaptive and stepwise changes in the rise and spread of antimicrobial resistance. In: Keen P, Monforts M, editors. Antimicrobial Resistance in the Environment. Hoboken, New Jersey, EUA: Wiley-Blackwell; 2011. pp. 43-71. ISBN: 978-1-118-15623-0

[6] Olivares J, Bernardini A, Garcia-Leon G, Corona F, Sanchez MB, Martinez JL. The intrinsic resistome of bacterial pathogens. Frontiers in Microbiology. 2013;**30**(4):103

[7] Lewis K, Shan Y. Persister Awakening. Molecular Cell. 2016;**63**(1):3-4

[8] Conlon BP, Rowe SE, Gandt AB, Nuxoll AS, Donegan NP, Zalis EA, et al. Persister formation in *Staphylococcus aureus* is associated with ATP depletion. Nature Microbiology. 2016;**1**:16051

[9] Shan Y, Brown Gandt A, Rowe SE, Deisinger JP, Conlon BP, Lewis K. ATP-dependent persister formation in *Escherichia coli*. MBio. 2017;**8**(1):e02267-e02216

[10] Magana M, Sereti C, Ioannidis A, Mitchell CA, Ball AR, Magiorkinis E, et al. Options and limitations in clinical investigation of bacterial biofilms. Clin Microbiol Ver. 2018;**31**(3):e00084-e00016

[11] Cameron DR, Shan Y, Zalis EA, Isabella V, Lewis K. A genetic determinant of persister cell formation in bacterial pathogens. Journal of Bacteriology. 2018;**200**(17):e00303-e00318

[12] Prestinaci F, Pezzotti P, Pantosti A. Antimicrobial resistance: A global, multifaceted phenomenon. Pathog Global Health. 2015;**109**(7):309-318

[13] Holmes AH, Moore LSP, Sundsfjord A, Steinbakk M, Regmi S, Karkey A, et al. Understanding the mechanisms and drivers of antimicrobial resistance. Lancet. 2016;**387**(10014):176-187

[14] Rice LB. Federal funding for the study of antimicrobial resistance in nosocomial pathogens: No ESKAPE. Infectious Diseases. 2008;**197**(8):1079-1081

[15] Friedman ND, Temkin E, Carmeli Y. The negative impact of antibiotic resistance. Clinical Microbiology and Infection. 2016;**22**(5):416

[16] Eze EC, Chenia HY, El Zowalaty ME. *Acinetobacter baumannii* biofilms: Effects of physicochemical factors, virulence, antibiotic resistance determinants, gene regulation, and future antimicrobial treatments. Infect Drug Resist. 2018;**15**(11):2277-2299

[17] Cosgaya C, Mari-Almirall M, van Assche A, Fernandez-Orth D, Mosqueda

N, Telli M, et al. *Acinetobacter dijkshoorniae* sp. nov., a member of the *Acinetobacter calcoaceticus-Acinetobacter baumannii* complex mainly recovered from clinical samples in different countries. International Journal of Systematic and Evolutionary Microbiology. 2016;**66**(10):4105-4111

[18] Nemec A, Krizova L, Maixnerova M, Sedo O, Brisse S, Higgins PG. *Acinetobacter seifertii* sp. nov., a member of the *Acinetobacter calcoaceticus-Acinetobacter baumannii* complex isolated from human clinical specimens. International Journal of Systematic and Evolutionary Microbiology. 2015; **63**(Pt 3):934-942

[19] Vijayakumar S, Biswas I, Veeraraghavan B. Accurate identification of clinically important *Acinetobacter spp.:* An update. Future Sci AO. 2019;**5**(6):FSO395

[20] Chen TL, Lee YT, Kuo SC, Yang SP, Fung CP, Lee SD. Rapid identification of *Acinetobacter baumannii, Acinetobacter nosocomialis*, and *Acinetobacter pittii* with a multiplex PCR assay. Journal of Medical Microbiology. 2014;**63**(Pt 9): 1154-1159

[21] Marí-Almirall M, Cosgaya C, Higgins PG, Van Assche A, Telli M, Huys G, et al. MALDI-TOF/MS identification of species from the *Acinetobacter baumannii* (ab) group revisited: Inclusion of the novel *a. seifertii* and *A. dijkshoorniae* species. Clinical Microbiology and Infection. 2017;**23**(3):210.e1-210.e9

[22] Peleg AY, Seifert H, Paterson DL. *Acinetobacter baumannii:* Emergence of a successful pathogen. Clinical Microbiology Reviews. 2008;**21**(3): 538-582

[23] Dijkshoorn L, Nemec A, Seifert H. An increasing threat in hospitals: Multidrug-resistant *Acinetobacter baumannii*. Nature Reviews. Microbiology. 2007;**5**(12):939-951

[24] Garnacho-Montero J, Timsit JF. Managing *Acinetobacter baumannii* infections. Current Opinion in Infectious Diseases. 2019;**32**(1):69-76

[25] Magiorakos AP, Srinivasan A, Carey RB, Carmeli Y, Falagas ME, Giske CG, et al. Multidrug-resistant, extensively drug-resistant and pan drug-resistant bacteria: An international expert proposal for interim standard definitions for acquired resistance. Clinical Microbiology and Infection. 2012;**18**(3):268-281

[26] Xie R, Zhang XD, Zhao Q, Peng B, Zheng J. Analysis of global prevalence of antibiotic resistance in *Acinetobacter baumannii* infections disclosed a faster increase in OECD countries. Emerg. Microb. Infect. 2018;**7**(1):1-10

[27] Willyard C. The drug-resistant bacteria that pose the greatest health threats. Nature. 2017;**543**(7643):15

[28] Barth VCJ, Rodrigues BÁ, Bonatto GD, Gallo SW, Pagnussatti VE, Ferreira CAS, et al. Heterogeneous persister cells formation in *Acinetobacter baumannii*. PLoS One. 2013;**8**(12):e84361

[29] Lukovic B, Gajic I, Dimkic I, Kekic D, Zornic S, Pozder T, et al. The first nationwide multicenter study of Acinetobacter baumannii recovered in Serbia: Emergence of OXA-72, OXA-23 and NDM-1-producing isolates. Antimicrobial Resistance and Infection Control. 2020;**9**(1):101

[30] Isler B, Doi Y, Bonomo RA, Paterson DL. New treatment options against carbapenem-resistant Acinetobacter baumannii infections. Antimicrobial Agents Chemother. 2019; **63**(1):e01110-e01118

[31] World Health Organization. Global priority list of antibiotic-resistant

bacteria to guide research, discovery, and development of new antibiotics. Available at: https://www.who.int/medicines/publications/WHO-PPL-Short_Summary_25Feb-ET_NM_WHO.pdf. [Accessed in July 2021]

[32] Domalaon R, Zhanel GG, Schweizer F. Short antimicrobial peptides and peptide scaffolds as promising antibacterial agents. Current Topics in Medicine Chemistry. 2016;**16**(11):1217-1230

[33] Vrancianu CO, Gheorghe I, Czobor IB, Chifiriuc MC. Antibiotic resistance profiles, molecular mechanisms, and innovative treatment strategies of *Acinetobacter baumannii*. Microorganisms. 2020;**8**(6):935

[34] Falanga A, Galdiero S. Emerging therapeutic agents on the basis of naturally occurring antimicrobial peptides. In: SPR, Amino Acids, Peptides and Proteins. Vol. 42. Cambridge, UK: Royal Society of Chemistry; 2018. pp. 190-227. ISBN: 978-1-78801-002-3

[35] Kang HK, Kim C, Seo CH, Park Y. The therapeutic applications of antimicrobial peptides (AMPs): A patent review. Journal of Microbiology. 2017;**55**(1):1-12

[36] Pasupuleti M, Schmidtchen A, Malmsten M. Antimicrobial peptides: Key components of the innate immune system. Critical Reviews in Biotechnology. 2012;**32**(2):143-171

[37] Wang G, Li X, Wang Z. APD3: The antimicrobial peptide database as a tool for research and education. Nucleic Acids Research. 2015;**44**(D1): D1087-D1093

[38] Neshani A, Zare H, Akbari Eidgahi MR, Chichaklu AH, Movaqar A, Ghazvini K. Review of antimicrobial peptides with anti-*helicobacter pylori* activity. Helicobacter. 2019;**24**(1): e12555

[39] Mansour SC, Pena OM, Hancock REW. Host defense peptides: front-line immunomodulators. Trends in Immunology. 2014;**35**(9):443-450

[40] Falanga A, Lombardi L, Franci G, Vitiello M, Iovene MR, Morelli G, et al. Marine antimicrobial peptides: Nature provides templates for the design of novel compounds against pathogenic bacteria. International Journal of Molecular Sciences. 2016;**17**(5):785

[41] Moretta A, Scieuzo C, Petrone AM, Salvia R, Manniello MD, Franco A, et al. Antimicrobial peptides: A new hope in biomedical and pharmaceutical fields. Frontiers in Cellular and Infection Microbiology. 2021;**11**:668632

[42] Haney EF, Brito-Sánchez Y, Trimble MJ, Mansour SC, Cherkasov A, Hancock REW. Computer-aided discovery of peptides that specifically attack bacterial biofilms. Scientific Reports. 2018;**8**(1): 1871

[43] Govender T, Dawood A, Esterhuyse AJ, Katerere DR. Antimicrobial properties of the skin secretions of frogs. South African Journal of Science. 2012;**108**:25-30

[44] Pfalzgraff A, Brandenburg K, Weindl G. Antimicrobial peptides and their therapeutic potential for bacterial skin infections and wounds. Frontiers in Pharmacology. 2018;**9**:281

[45] Neshani A, Zare H, Akbari Eidgahi MR, Khaledi A, Ghazvini K. Epinecidin-1, a highly potent marine antimicrobial peptide with anticancer and immunomodulatory activities. BMC. Pharmacology & Toxicology. 2019; **20**(1):33. DOI: 10.1186/s40360-019-0309-7

[46] Neshani A, Tanhaeian A, Zare H, Eidgahi MRA, Ghazvini K. Preparation and evaluation of a new biopesticide solution candidate for plant disease

control using pexiganan gene and Pichia pastoris expression system. Gene Rep. 2019;**17**:100509

[47] Fan L, Sun J, Zhou M, Zhou J, Lao X, Zheng H. DRAMP: A comprehensive data repository of antimicrobial peptides. Scientific Reports. 2016;**14**(6): 24482

[48] Kumar P, Kizhakkedathu JN, Straus SK. Antimicrobial peptides: Diversity, mechanism of action, and strategies to improve the activity and biocompatibility in vivo. Biomolecules. 2018;**8**(1):4

[49] Zhang LJ, Gallo RL. Antimicrobial peptides. Current Biology. 2016;**26**(1): R14-R19

[50] Zhang G, Sunkara LT. Avian antimicrobial host defense peptides: From biology to therapeutic applications. Pharmaceuticals. 2014;**7** (3):220

[51] Cruz J, Ortiz C, Guzman F, Fernandez-Lafuente R, Torres R. Antimicrobial peptides: Promising compounds against pathogenic microorganisms. Current Medicinal Chemistry. 2014;**21**(20):2299

[52] Epand RM, Walker C, Epand RF, Magarvey NA. Molecular mechanisms of membrane targeting antibiotics. Biochimica et Biophysica Acta - Biomembranes. 2016;**1858**:980-987

[53] Andersson DI, Hughes D, Kubicek-Sutherland JZ. Mechanisms and consequences of bacterial resistance to antimicrobial peptides. Drug Resist. Updated. 2016;**26**:43-57

[54] Ehrenstein G, Lecar H. Electrically gated ionic channels in lipid bilayers. Quarterly Reviews of Biophysics. 1977; **10**:1-34

[55] Brogden KA. Antimicrobial peptides: Pore formers or metabolic inhibitors in bacteria? Nature Reviews. Microbiology. 2005;**3**:238-250

[56] Breukink E, de Kruijff B. The lantibiotic nisin, a special case or not? Biochimica et Biophysica Acta. 1999; **1462**:223-234

[57] Wimley WC. Describing the mechanism of antimicrobial peptide action with the interfacial activity model. ACS Chemical Biology. 2010;**5**: 905-917

[58] Rapaport D, Shai Y. Interaction of fluorescently labeled pardaxin and its analogs with lipid bilayers. The Journal of Biological Chemistry. 1991;**266**: 23769-23775

[59] Shai Y, Bach D, Yanovsky A. Channel formation properties of synthetic pardaxin and analogs. The Journal of Biological Chemistry. 1990; **265**:20202-20209

[60] Uematsu N, Matsuzaki K. Polar angle as a determinant of amphipathic α-helix-lipid interactions: A model peptide study. Biophysical Journal. 2000;**79**:2075-2083

[61] Yeaman MR, Yount NY. Mechanisms of antimicrobial peptide action and resistance. Pharmacological Reviews. 2003;**55**:27-55

[62] Lee T-H, Hall KN, Aguilar M-I. Antimicrobial peptide structure and mechanism of action: A focus on the role of membrane structure. Current Topics in Medicinal Chemistry. 2016;**16**:25-39

[63] Cheng JTJ, Hale JD, Elliot M, Hancock REW, Straus SK. Effect of membrane composition on antimicrobial peptides aurein 2.2 and 2.3 from Australian southern bell frogs. Biophysical Journal. 2009;**96**:552-565

[64] Sparr E, Ash WL, Nazarov PV, Rijkers DTS, Hemminga MA, Tieleman DP, et al. Self-association of

transmembrane-helices in model membranes. The Journal of Biological Chemistry. 2005;**280**:39324-39331

[65] Cheng JTJ, Hale JD, Elliott M, Hancock REW, Straus SK. The importance of bacterial membrane composition in the structure and function of aurein 2.2 and selected variants. Biochimica et Biophysica Acta - Biomembranes. 2011;**1808**:622-633

[66] Shai Y. Mode of action of membrane-active antimicrobial peptides. Biopolymers. 2002;**66**:236-248

[67] Fernandez DI, Le Brun AP, Whitwell TC, Sani M-A, James M, Separovic F. The antimicrobial peptide aurein 1.2 disrupts model membranes via the carpet mechanism. Physical Chemistry Chemical Physics. 2012;**14**: 15739

[68] Sitaram N, Nagaraj R. Interaction of antimicrobial peptides with biological and model membranes: Structural and charge requirements for activity. Biochimica et Biophysica Acta. 1999; **1462**:29-54

[69] Rozek A, Friedrich CL, Hancock RE. Structure of the bovine antimicrobial peptide indolicidin bound to dodecyl phosphocholine and sodium dodecyl sulfate micelles. Biochemistry. 2000;**39**: 15765-15774

[70] Gee ML, Burton M, Grevis-James A, Hossain MA, McArthur S, Palombo EA, et al. Imaging the action of antimicrobial peptides on living bacterial cells. Scientific Reports. 2013;**3**:1557

[71] Choi H, Rangarajan N, Weisshaar JC. Lights, camera, action! Antimicrobial peptide mechanisms imaging in space and time. Trends in Microbiology. 2016;**24**:111-122

[72] Manzini MC, Perez KR, Riske KA, Bozelli JC, Santos TL, da Silva MA, et al. Peptide: Lipid ratio and membrane surface charge determine the mechanism of action of the antimicrobial peptide BP100. Conformational and functional studies. Biochimica et Biophysica Acta - Biomembranes. 2014;**1838**:1985-1999

[73] Feng X, Sambanthamoorthy K, Palys T, Paranavitana C. The human antimicrobial peptide LL-37 and its fragments possess both antimicrobial and antibiofilm activities against multidrug-resistant *Acinetobacter baumannii*. Peptides. 2013;**49**:131-137

[74] de Breij A, Riool M, Cordfunke RA, Malanovic N, de Boer L, Koning RI, et al. The antimicrobial peptide SAAP-148 combats drug-resistant bacteria and biofilms. Sci Transl. 2018;**10**(423): eaan4044

[75] Tajbakhsh M, Akhavan MM, Fallah F, Karimi A. A recombinant snake cathelicidin derivative peptide: Antibiofilm properties and expression in *Escherichia Coli*. Biomolecules. 2018;**8**(4):118

[76] Mwangi J, Yin Y, Wang G, Yang M, Li Y, Zhang Z, et al. The antimicrobial peptide ZY4 combats multidrug-resistant *Pseudomonas aeruginosa* and *Acinetobacter baumannii* Infection. Proc Natl Acad Sci. USA. 2019;**116**(52): 26516-26522

[77] Barksdale SM, Hrifko EJ, van Hoek ML. Cathelicidin antimicrobial peptide from Alligator mississippiensis has antibacterial activity against multi-drug resistant Acinetobacter baumanii and Klebsiella pneumoniae. Developmental and Comparative Immunology. 2017;**70**: 135-144

[78] Zhao F, Lan XQ, Du Y, Chen PY, Zhao J, Zhao F, et al. King cobra peptide OH-CATH30 as a potential candidate drug through clinic drug-resistant isolates. Zoological Research. 2018; **39**(2):87-96

[79] Dekan Z, Headey SJ, Scanlon M, Baldo BA, Lee TH, Aguilar MI, et al. Δ-Myrtoxin-Mp1a is a helical heterodimer from the venom of the jack jumper ant that has antimicrobial, membrane-disrupting, and nociceptive activities. Angewandte Chemie (International Ed. in English). 2017;**56** (29):8495-8499

[80] Al-Asmari AK, Alamri MA, Almasoudi AS, Abbasmanthiri R, Mahfoud M. Evaluation of the in vitro antimicrobial activity of selected Saudi scorpion venoms tested against multidrug-resistant micro-organisms. J Glob Antimicrob Resist. 2017;**10**:14-18

[81] Domhan C, Uhl P, Kleist C, Zimmermann S, Umstätter F, Leotta K, et al. Replacement of L-amino acids by d-amino acids in the antimicrobial peptide ranalexin and its consequences for antimicrobial activity and biodistribution. Molecules. 2019;**24**(16): 2987

[82] Hirsch R, Wiesner J, Marker A, Pfeifer Y, Bauer A, Hammann PE, et al. Profiling antimicrobial peptides from the medical maggot Lucilia sericata as potential antibiotics for MDR gram-negative bacteria. The Journal of Antimicrobial Chemotherapy. 2019;**74** (1):96-107

[83] Shamova OV, Orlov DS, Zharkova MS, Balandin SV, Yamschikova EV, Knappe D, et al. Minibactenecins ChBac7.Nα and ChBac7. Nβ—Antimicrobial peptides from leukocytes of the goat *Capra hircus*. Acta Naturae. 2016;**8**(3):136-146

[84] Spencer JJ, Pitts RE, Pearson RA, King LB. The effects of antimicrobial peptides WAM-1 and LL-37 on multidrug-resistant Acinetobacter baumannii. Pathogens and Disease. 2018;**76**(2):fty007

[85] Vila-Farres X, De La Maria CG, López-Rojas R, Pachón J, Giralt E, Vila J. In vitro activity of several antimicrobial peptides against colistin-susceptible and colistin-resistant *Acinetobacter baumannii*. Clinical Microbiology and Infection. 2012;**18**(4):383-387

[86] Giacometti A, Cirioni O, Del Prete MS, Barchiesi F, Paggi AM, Petrelli E, et al. Comparative activities of polycationic peptides and clinically used antimicrobial agents against multidrug-resistant nosocomial isolates of *Acinetobacter baumannii*. The Journal of Antimicrobial Chemotherapy. 2000; **46**(5):807-810

[87] Falla TJ, Karunaratne DN, Hancock RE. Mode of action of the antimicrobial peptide indolicidin. The Journal of Biological Chemistry. 1996;**271**(32): 19298-19303

[88] Romeo D, Skerlavaj B, Bolognesi M, Gennaro R. Structure and bactericidal activity of an antibiotic dodecapeptide purified from bovine neutrophils. The Journal of Biological Chemistry. 1988; **263**(20):9573-9575

[89] Wu M, Hancock RE. Interaction of the cyclic antimicrobial cationic peptide bactenecin with the outer and cytoplasmic membrane. The Journal of Biological Chemistry. 1999;**274**(1):29-35

[90] Skerlavaj B, Romeo D, Gennaro R. Rapid membrane permeabilization and inhibition of vital functions of gram-negative bacteria by bactenecins. Infection and Immunity. 1990;**58**(11): 3724-3730

[91] Shamova O, Orlov D, Stegemann C, Czihal P, Hoffmann R, Brogden K, et al. ChBac34: A novel proline-rich antimicrobial peptide from goat leukocytes. Int J Pept Res Therapy. 2009;**15**(1):31-42

[92] Seefeldt AC, Graf M, Pérébaskine N, Nguyen F, Arenz S, Mardirossian M, et al. Structure of the mammalian

antimicrobial peptide Bac7(1-16) bound within the exit tunnel of a bacterial ribosome. Nucleic Acids Research. 2016; **44**(5):2429-2438

[93] Wang C, Zhao G, Wang S, Chen Y, Gong Y, Chen S, et al. A simplified derivative of human defensin 5 with potent and efficient activity against multidrug-resistant *Acinetobacter baumannii*. Antimicrobial Agents and Chemotherapy. 2018;**62**(2):e01504-e01517

[94] Kaushal A, Gupta K, van Hoek ML. Characterization of *Cimex lectularius* (bedbug) defensin peptide and its antimicrobial activity against human skin microflora. Biochemical and Biophysical Research Communications. 2016;**470**(4):955-960

[95] Routsias JG, Karagounis P, Parvulesku G, Legakis NJ, Tsakris A. In vitro bactericidal activity of human β-defensin 2 against nosocomial strains. Peptides. 2010;**31**(9):1654-1660

[96] Maisetta G, Batoni G, Esin S, Florio W, Bottai D, Favilli F, et al. In vitro bactericidal activity of human beta-defensin 3 against multidrug-resistant nosocomial strains. Antimicrobial Agents and Chemotherapy. 2006;**50**(2):806-809

[97] Kim MK, Kang N, Ko SJ, Park J, Park E, Shin DW, et al. Antibacterial and antibiofilm activity and mode of action of magainin 2 against drug-resistant *Acinetobacter baumannii*. International Journal of Molecular Sciences. 2018;**19**(10):3041

[98] Zasloff M. Magainins a class of antimicrobial peptides from Xenopus skin: Isolation characterization of two active forms and partial cDNA sequence of a precursor. Proc Natl Acad Sci USA. 1987;**84**(15):5449-5453

[99] Flamm RK, Rhomberg PR, Simpson KM, Farrell DJ, Sader HS, Jones RN. In vitro spectrum of pexiganan activity when tested against pathogens from diabetic oot infections and with selected resistance mechanisms. Antimicrobial Agents and Chemotherapy. 2015;**59**(3): 1751-1754

[100] Ge Y MacDonald, DL Holroyd, KJ Thornsberry C, Wexler H, Zasloff M. In vitro antibacterial properties of pexiganan an analog of magainin. Antimicrobial Agents and Chemotherapy 1999; 43(4):782-788.

[101] Jáskiewicz M, Neubauer D, Kazor K, Bartoszewska S, Kamysz W. Antimicrobial activity of selected antimicrobial peptides against planktonic culture and biofilm of *Acinetobacter baumannii*. Probiotics Antimicrob Proteins. 2019;**11**(1):317-324

[102] Conlon JM, Ahmed E, Condamine E. Antimicrobial properties of brevinin-2-related peptide and its analogs: Efficacy against multidrug-resistant *Acinetobacter baumannii*. Chemical Biology & Drug Design. 2009;**74**(5):488-493

[103] Conlon JM, Sonnevend A, Pál T, Vila-Farrés X. Efficacy of six frog skin-derived antimicrobial peptides against colistin-resistant strains of the *Acinetobacter baumannii* group. International Journal of Antimicrobial Agents. 2012;**39**(4):317-320

[104] Liu CB, Shan B, Bai HM, Tang J, Yan LZ, Ma YB. Hydrophilic/ hydrophobic characters of antimicrobial peptides derived from animals and their effects on multidrug-resistant clinical isolates. Dongwuxue Yanjiu = Zool Res. 2015;**36**(1):41-47

[105] Al-Ghaferi N, Kolodziejek J, Nowotny N, Coquet L, Jouenne T, Leprince J, et al. Antimicrobial peptides from the skin secretions of the southeast Asian frog *Hylarana erythraea* (*Ranidae*). Peptides. 2010;**31**(4):548-554

[106] Conlon JM, Ahmed E, Pal T. A Sonnevend potent and rapid bactericidal

action of alyteserin-1c and its [E4K] analog against multidrug-resistant strains of *Acinetobacter baumannii*. Peptides. 2010;**31**(10):1806-1810

[107] Conlon JM, Mechkarska M, Arafat K, Attoub S, Sonnevend A. Analogues of the frog skin peptide alyteserin-2a with enhanced antimicrobial activities against gram-negative bactéria. Journal of Peptide Science. 2012;**18**(4):270-275

[108] McLean DTF, McCrudden MTC, Linden GJ, Irwin CR, Conlon JM, Lundy FT. Antimicrobial and immunomodulatory properties of PGLa-AM1 CPFAM1 and magainin-AM1: Potent activity against oral pathogens. Regulatory Peptides. 2014;**194-195**:63-68

[109] Conlon JM, Al-Ghaferi N, Ahmed E, Meetani MA, Leprince JJ, Nielsen PF. Orthologs of magainin PGLa procaerulein-derived and proxenopsin-derived peptides from skin secretions of the octoploid frog *Xenopus amieti* (*Pipidae*). Peptides. 2010;**31**(6):989-994

[110] Conlon JM, Mechkarska M, Ahmed E, Leprince J, Vaudry H, King JD, et al. Purification and properties of antimicrobial peptides from skin secretions of the Eritrea clawed frog *Xenopus clivii* (*Pipidae*). Comp Biochem Physiol C Toxicol Pharmacol. 2011;**153** (3):350-354

[111] Mechkarska M, Ahmed E, Coquet L, Leprince J, Jouenne T, Vaudry H, et al. Antimicrobial peptides with therapeutic potential from skin secretions of the Marsabit clawed frog *Xenopus borealis* (*Pipidae*). Comp Biochem Physiol C Toxicol Pharmacol. 2010;**152**(4):467-472

[112] Mechkarska M, Prajeep M, Radosavljevic GD, Jovanovic IP, Al Baloushi A, Sonnevend A, et al. An analog of the host-defense peptide hymenochirin-1B with potent broad-spectrum activity against multidrug-resistant bacteria and immunomodulatory properties. Peptides. 2013;**50**:153-159

[113] Serra I, Scorciapino MA, Manzo G, Casu M, Rinaldi AC, Attoub S, et al. Conformational analysis and cytotoxic activities of the frog skin host-defense peptide hymenochirin-1Pa. Peptides. 2014;**61**:114-121

[114] Conlon JM, Galadari S, Raza H, Condamine E. Design of potent non-toxic antimicrobial agents based upon the naturally occurring frog skin peptides ascaphin-8 and peptide XT-7. Chemical Biology & Drug Design. 2008;**72**(1):58-64

[115] Park CB, Kim HS, Kim SC. Mechanism of action of the antimicrobial peptide buforin II: Buforin II kills microorganisms by penetrating the cell membrane and inhibiting cellular functions. Biochemical and Biophysical Research Communications. 1998;**244**(1):253-257

[116] Cirioni O, Silvestri C, Ghiselli R, Orlando F, Riva A, Gabrielli E, et al. Therapeutic efficacy of buforin II and rifampin in a rat model of *Acinetobacter baumannii* sepsis. Critical Care Medicine. 2009;**37**(4):1403-1407

[117] Pashaei F, Bevalian P, Akbari R, Bagheri KP. Single-dose eradication of extensively drug-resistant *Acinetobacter* spp. in a mouse model of burn infection by melittin antimicrobial peptide. Microbial Pathogenesis. 2019;**127**:60-69

[118] Akbari R, Hakemi-Vala M, Pashaie F, Bevalian P, Hashemi A, Bagheri KP. Highly synergistic effects of melittin with conventional antibiotics against multidrug-resistant isolates of *Acinetobacter baumannii* and *Pseudomonas aeruginosa*. Microbial Drug Resistance. 2019;**25**(2):193-202

[119] Giacometti A, Cirioni O, Kamysz W, D'Amato G, Silvestri C, Del Prete MS, et al. Comparative activities of

cecropin a melittin and cecropin A-melittin peptide CA(1-7)M(2-9)NH2 against multidrug-resistant nosocomial isolates of *Acinetobacter baumannii*. Peptides. 2003;**24**(9):1315-1318

[120] Jayamani E, Rajamuthiah R, Larkins-Ford J, Fuchs BB, Conery AL, Vilcinskas A, et al. Insect-derived cecropins display activity against *Acinetobacter baumannii* in a whole-animal high-throughput *Caenorhabditis elegans* model. Antimicrobial Agents and Chemotherapy. 2015;**59**(3):1728-1737

[121] Gui S, Li R, Feng Y, Wang S. Transmission electron microscopic morphological study and flow cytometric viability assessment of *Acinetobacter baumannii* susceptible to *Musca domestica* cecropin. Scientific World Journal. 2014;**2014**:657536

[122] Boman HG, Agerberth B, Boman A. Mechanisms of action on *Escherichia coli* of cecropin P1 and PR-39 two antibacterial peptides from pig intestine. Infection and Immunity. 1993;**61**(7):2978-2984

[123] Peng J, Long H, Liu W, Wu Z, Wang T, Zeng Z, et al. Antibacterial mechanism of peptide cec4 against *Acinetobacter baumannii*. Infect Drug Resist. 2019;**12**:2417-2428

[124] Han HM, Ko S, Cheong M-J, Bang JK, Seo CH, Luchian T, et al. Myxinidin2 and myxinidin3 suppress inflammatory responses through STAT3 and MAPKs to promote wound healing. Oncotarget. 2017;**8**(50):87582-87597

[125] Gordya N, Yakovlev A, Kruglikova A, Tulin D, Potolitsina E, Suborova T, et al. Natural antimicrobial peptide complexes in the fighting of antibiotic-resistant biofilms: *Calliphora vicina* medicinal maggots. PLoS One. 2017;**12**(3):e0173559

[126] Vila-Farrés X, López-Rojas R, Pachón-Ibáñez ME, Teixidó M, Pachón J, Vila J, et al. Sequence-activity relationship and mechanism of action of mastoparan analogues against extended-drug resistant *Acinetobacter baumannii*. European Journal of Medicinal Chemistry. 2015;**101**:34-40

[127] Al-Khafaji Z, Al-Samaree M. Design of synthetic antimicrobial peptides against resistant *Acinetobacter baumannii* using computational approach. Int J Pharmaceut Sci Res. 2017;**8**:2033-2039255

[128] Lin CH, Lee MC, Tzen JTC, Lee HM, Chang SM, Tu WC, et al. Efficacy of mastoparan-AF alone and in combination with clinically used antibiotics on nosocomial multidrug-resistant *Acinetobacter baumannii* Saudi. Journal of Biological Sciences. 2017;**24**(5):1023-1029

[129] Tartar AS, Balın SO, Akbulut A, Yardım M, Aydın S. Roles of Dermcidin Salusin-α Salusin-β and TNF-α in the pathogenesis of human brucellosis. Iranian Journal of Immunology. 2019;**16**(2):182-189

[130] Farshadzadeh Z, Modaresi MH, Taheri B, Rahimi S, Bahador A. InVitro antimicrobial activity of dermcidin-1L against extensively-drug-resistant and pandrug resistant *Acinetobacter baumannii*. Jundishapur J Microbiol. 2017;**10**(5):e13201

[131] Mohamed MF, Hamed MI, Panitch A, Seleem MN. Targeting methicillin-resistant *Staphylococcus aureus* with short salt-resistant synthetic peptides. Antimicrobial Agents and Chemotherapy. 2014;**58**(7):4113-4122

[132] Mohamed MF, Brezden A, Mohammad H, Chmielewski J, Seleem MN. A short D-enantiomeric antimicrobial peptide with potent immunomodulatory and antibiofilm activity against multidrug-resistant *Pseudomonas aeruginosa* and *Acinetobacter baumannii*. Scientific Reports. 2017;7(1):6953

[133] Wu X, Li Z, Li X, Tian Y, Fan Y, Yu C, et al. Synergistic effects of antimicrobial peptide DP7 combined with antibiotics against multidrug-resistant bacteria. Drug Des Dev Ther. 2017;**11**:939-946

[134] Zhang R, Wang Z, Tian Y, Yin Q, Cheng X, Lian M, et al. Efficacy of antimicrobial peptide DP7 designed by machine-learning method against methicillin-resistant *Staphylococcus aureus*. Frontiers in Microbiology. 2019;**10**:1175

[135] Nagarajan D, Roy N, Kulkarni O, Nanajkar N, Datey A, Ravichandran S, et al. Ω76: A designed antimicrobial peptide to combat carbapenem- and tigecycline resistant *Acinetobacter baumannii*. Science Advances. 2019;**5**(7):eaax1946

[136] Mourtada R, Herce HD, Yin DJ, Moroco JÁ, Wales TE, Engen JR, et al. Design of stapled antimicrobial peptides that are stable, nontoxic, and kill antibiotic-resistant bacteria in mice. Nature Biotechnology. 2019;**37**(10): 1186-1197

[137] Rose M, Lapuebla A, Landman D, Quale J. In vitro and in vivo activity of a novel antisense peptide nucleic acid compound against multidrug-resistant *Acinetobacter baumannii*. Microbial Drug Resistance. 2019;**25**(7):961-965

[138] Gopal R, Kim YG, Lee JH, Lee SK, Chae JD, Son BK, et al. Synergistic effects and antibiofilm properties of chimeric peptides against multidrug-resistant Acinetobacter baumannii strains. Antimicrobial Agents and Chemotherapy. 2014;**58**(3):1622-1629

[139] Hong MJ, Kim MK, Park Y. Compa rative antimicrobial activity of Hp404 peptide and its analogs against *Acine tobacter baumannii*. International Journal of Molecular Sciences. 2021; **22**(11):5540

[140] Neshani A, Sedighian H, Mirhosseini SA, Ghazvini K, Zare H, Jahangiri A. Antimicrobial peptides as a promising treatment option against Acinetobacter baumannii infections. Microbial Pathogenesis. 2020;**146**:104238

[141] Jayathilaka EHTT, Rajapaksha DC, Nikapitiya C, De Zoysa M, Whang I. Antimicrobial and anti-biofilm peptide octominin for controlling multidrug-re sistant *Acinetobacter baumannii*. International Journal of Molecular Sciences. 2021;**22**(10):5353

[142] Hacioglu M, Oyardi O, Bozkurt-Guzel C, Savage PB. Antibiofilm activities of ceragenins and antimicrobial peptides against fungal-bacterial mono and multispecies biofilms. Journal of Antibiotics (Tokyo). 2020;**73**(7):455-462

[143] Morroni G, Simonetti O, Brenciani A, Brescini L, Kamysz W, Kamysz E, et al. In vitro activity of protegrin-1 alone and in combination with clinically useful antibiotics against *Acinetobacter baumannii* strains isolated from surgical wounds. Medical Microbiology and Immunology. 2019;**208**(6):877-883

[144] Sharma D, Choudhary M, Vashistt J, Shrivastava R, SinghBisht G. Cationic antimicrobial peptide and its poly-N-substituted glycine congener: Antibacterial and antibiofilm potential against *a baumannii*. Biochemical and Biophysical Research Communications. 2019;**518**(3):472-478

[145] Mohan NM, Zorgani A, Jalowicki G, Kerr A, Khaldi N, Martins M. Unlocking nuripep 1653 from common pea protein: A potent antimicrobial peptide to tackle a pan-drug resistant *Acinetobacter baumannii*. Frontiers in Microbiology. 2019;**10**:2086

[146] Dowzinkly MJ, Chmelarová E. Antimicrobial susceptibility of gram-negative and gram-positive bacteria collected from Eastern Europe: Results from the Tigecycline evaluation and surveillance trial (T.E.S>T.), 2011-2016.

J. Glob. Antimicrobial Resist. 2019; **17**(44):44-52. DOI: 10.1016/j. jgar.2018.11.007

[147] Björstad Å, Askarieh G, Brown KL, Christenson K, Forsman H, Önnheim K, et al. The host defense peptide LL-37 selectively permeabilizes apoptotic leukocytes. Antimicrob Ag Chemother. 2009;**53**(3):1027-1038. DOI: 10.1128/ AAC.01310-08

[148] De Y, Chen Q, Schmidt AP, Anderson GM, Wang JM, Wooters J, et al. LL-37 the neutrophil granule-and epithelial cell-derived cathelicidin utilizes formyl peptide receptor-like 1 (FPRL1) as a receptor to chemoattract human peripheral blood neutrophils monocytes and T cells. The Journal of Experimental Medicine. 2000;**192**(7):1069-1074. DOI: 10.1084/jem.192.7.1069

[149] Nijnik A, Hancock REW. Host defense peptides: Antimicrobial and immunomodulatory activity and potential applications for tackling antibiotic-resistant infections. Emerg. Health Threats J. 2009;**2**:e1. DOI: 10.3134/ehtj.09.001

[150] Neshani A, Zare H, Eidgahi MRA, Kakhki RK, Safdari H, Khaledi A, et al. LL-37: A review of antimicrobial profile against sensitive and antibiotic-resistant human bacterial pathogens. Gene Rep. 2019;**17**:100519. DOI: 10.1016/j.genrep. 2019.100519

[151] Esfandiyari R, Halabian R, Behzadi E, Sedighian H, Jafari R, Fooladi AAI. Performance evaluation of antimicrobial peptide ll-37 and hepcidin and β-defensin-2 secreted by mesenchymal stem cells. Heliyon. 2019;**5**(10):e02652. DOI: 10.1016/j.heliyon.2019.e02652

[152] Liu C, Shan B, Qi J, Ma Y. Systemic responses of multidrug-resistant *Pseudomonas aeruginosa* and *Acinetobacter baumannii* following exposure to the antimicrobial peptide cathelicidin-BF imply multiple intracellular targets. Frontiers in Cellular and Infection Microbiology. 2017;**7**:466. DOI: 10.3389/fcimb. 2017.00466

[153] Zhao H, Gan TX, Liu XD, Jin Y, Lee WH, Shen JH, et al. Identification and characterization of novel reptile cathelicidins from elapid snakes. Peptides. 2008;**29**(10):1685-1691. DOI: 10.1016/j.peptides.2008.06.008

[154] Du H, Samuel RL, Massiah MA, Gillmor SD. The structure and behavior of the NA-CATH antimicrobial peptide with liposomes. Biochimica et Biophysica Acta. 2015;**1848**(10 Pt A): 2394-2405. DOI: 10.1016/j.bbamem. 2015.07.006

[155] Ikenaga M, Guevara R, Dean AL, Pisani C, Boyer JN. Changes in community structure of sediment bacteria along the Florida coastal everglades marsh-mangrove-seagrass salinity gradient. Microbial Ecology. 2010;**59**(2):284-295. DOI: 10.1007/ s00248-009-9572-2

[156] Bishop BM, Juba ML, Devine MC, Barksdale SM, Rodriguez CA, Chung MC, et al. Bioprospecting the American alligator (*Alligator mississippiensis*) host defense peptidome. PLoS One. 2015;**10** (2):e0117394. DOI: 10.1371/journal. pone.0117394

[157] Daly KA, Digby MR, Lefévre C, Nicholas KR, Deane EM, Williamson P. Identification characterization and expression of cathelicidin in the pouch young of Tammar wallaby (*Macropus eugenii*). Comparative Biochemistry and Physiology. Part B, Biochemistry & Molecular Biology. 2008;**149**(3): 524-533. DOI: 10.1016/j. cbpb.2007.12.002

[158] Selsted ME, Novotny MJ, Morris WL, Tang YQ, Smith W, Cullor JS. Indolicidin is a novel bactericidal tridecapeptide amide from neutrophils.

The Journal of Biological Chemistry. 1992;**267**(7):4292-4295

[159] Végh AG, Nagy K, Bálint Z, Kerényi A, Rákhely G, Váró G, et al. Effect of antimicrobial peptide-amide: Indolicidin on biological membranes. Journal of Biomedicine & Biotechnology. 2011;**2011**:670589. DOI: 10.1155/2011/670589

[160] Hsu CH, Chen C, Jou ML, Lee AYL, Lin YC, Yu YP, et al. Structural and DNA-binding studies on the bovine antimicrobial peptide indolicidin: Evidence for multiple conformations involved in binding to membranes and DNA. Nucleic Acids Research. 2005; **33**(13):4053-4064. DOI: 10.1093/nar/gki725

[161] Marchand C, Krajewski K, Lee HF, Antony S, Johnson AA, Amin R, et al. Covalent binding of the natural antimicrobial peptide indolicidin to DNA abasic sites. Nucleic Acids Research. 2006;**34**(18):5157-5165. DOI: 10.1093/nar/gkl667

[162] Schneider JJ, Unholzer A, Schaller M, Schäfer-Korting M, Korting HC. Human defensins, Journal of Molecular Medicine (Berlin, Germany). 2005; **83**(8):587-595. DOI: 10.1007/s00109-005-0657-1

[163] Knutelski S, Awad M, Łukasz N, Bukowski M, Śmiałek J, Suder P, et al. Isolation, identification, and bioinformatic analysis of antibacterial proteins and peptides from immunized hemolymph of red palm weevil Rhynchophorus ferrugineus. Biomolecules. 2021;**11**(1):83. DOI: 10.3390/ iom11010083

[164] Lehrer RI, Lu W. α-Defensins in human innate immunity. Immunological Reviews. 2012;**45**(1):84-112. DOI: 10.1111/j.1600-065X.2011.01082.x

[165] Wang C, Zhao G, Wang S, Chen Y, Gong Y, Chen S, et al. A simplified derivative of human defensin 5 with potent and efficient activity against multidrug-resistant *Acinetobacter baumannii*. Antimicrobial Agents and Chemotherapy. 2018;**62**(2):e01504-e01517. DOI: 10.1128/AAC.01504-17

[166] Wanniarachchi YA, Kaczmarek P, Wan A, Nolan EM. Human defensin 5 disulfide array mutants: Disulfide bond deletion attenuates antibacterial activity against *Staphylococcus aureus*. Biochemistry. 2011;**37**:8005-8017. DOI: 10.1021/bi201043j

[167] Marcelino-Pérez G, Ruiz-Medrano R, Gallardo-Hernández S, Xoconostle-Cázares B. Adsorption of recombinant human β-defensin 2 and two mutants on mesoporous silica nanoparticles and its effect against *Clavibacter michiganensis* subsp. Michiganensis. Nanomaterials (Basel). 2021;**11**(8):2144. DOI: 10.3390/nano11082144

[168] Hirsch T, Spielmann M, Zuhaili B, Fossum M, Metzig M, Koehler T, et al. Human beta defensin-3 promotes wound healing in infected diabetic wounds. The Journal of Gene Medicine. 2009;**11**(3): 220-228. DOI: 10.1002/jgm.1287

[169] Zerweck J, Strandberg E, Kukharenko O, Reichert J, Bürck J, Wadhwani P, et al. Molecular mechanism of synergy between the antimicrobial peptides PGLa and magainin 2. Scientific Reports. 2017;**7**: 13153. DOI: 10.1038/s41598-017-12599-7

[170] Tamba Y, Yamazaki M. Magainin 2-induced pore formation in the lipid membranes depends on its concentration in the membrane interface. The Journal of Physical Chemistry. B. 2009;**113**(14):4846-4852. DOI: 10.1021/jp8109622

[171] Maloy WL, Kari UP. Structure-activity studies on magainins and other host defense peptides. Biopolymers. 1995;**37**(2):105-122. DOI: 10.1002/bip.360370206

[172] Gottler LM, Ramamoorthy A. Structure membrane orientation mechanism and function of pexiganan-a highly potent antimicrobial peptide designed from magainin. Biochimica et Biophysica Acta. 2009;**1788**(8):1680-1686

[173] Ramamoorthy A, Thennarasu S, Lee DK, Tan A, Maloy L. Solid-state NMR investigation of the membrane-disrupting mechanism of antimicrobial peptides MSI-78 and MSI-594 derived from magainin 2 and melittin. Biophysical Journal. 2006;**91**(1):206-216. DOI: 10.1529/biophysj.105.07 3890

[174] Fuchs PC, Barry AL, Brown SD. *In vitro* antimicrobial activity of MSI-78 a magainin analog. Antimicrobial Agents and Chemotherapy. 1998;**42**(5):1213-1216. DOI: 10.1128/AAC. 42.5.1213

[175] Bevier CR, Sonnevend A, Kolodziejek J, Nowotny N, Nielsen PF, Conlon JM. Purification and characterization of antimicrobial peptides from the skin secretions of the mink frog (*Rana septentrionalis*). Comp. Biochem. Physiol. C. Toxicol. Pharmacol. 2004;**139**(1–3):31-38. DOI: 10.1016/j.cca.2004.08.019

[176] Conlon JM, Abraham B, Sonnevend A, Jouenne T, Cosette P, Leprince J, et al. Purification and characterization of antimicrobial peptides from the skin secretions of the carpenter frog *Rana virgatipes* (Ranidae, Aquarana). Regulatory Peptides. 2005;**131**(1–3):38-45. DOI: 10.1016/j.regpep.20 05.06.003

[177] Savelyeva A, Ghavami S, Davoodpour P, Asoodeh A, Los MJ. An overview of Brevinin superfamily: Structure function and clinical perspectives. Advances in Experimental Medicine and Biology. 2014;**818**:197-212. DOI: 10.1007/978-1-4471-6458-610

[178] Popovic S, Urbán E, Lukic M, Conlon JM. Peptides with antimicrobial and anti-inflammatory activities that have therapeutic potential for treatment of acne vulgaris. Peptides. 2012;**34**(2): 275-282. DOI: 10.1016/j.peptides.2012. 02.010

[179] Popovic S, Djurdjevic P, Zaric M, Mijailovic Z, Avramovic D, Baskic D. Effects of host defense peptides B2RP Brevinin-2GU D-Lys-Temporin Lys-XT-7 and DLys-Ascaphin-8 on peripheral blood mononuclear cells: Preliminary study. Periodicum Biologorum. 2017;**119**(2):113-118. DOI: 10.18054/pb.v119i2.4781

[180] Conlon JM, Demandt A, Nielsen PF, Leprince J, Vaudry H, Woodhams DC. The alyteserins: Two families of antimicrobial peptides from the skin secretions of the midwife toad *Alytes obstetricans* (*Alytidae*). Peptides. 2009; **30**(6):1069-1073. DOI: 10.1016/ j.peptides.2009.03.004

[181] Subasinghage AP, O'Flynn D, Conlon JM, Hewage CM. Conformational and membrane interaction studies of the antimicrobial peptide alyteserin-1c and its analog [E4K] alyteserin-1c. Biochimica et Biophysica Acta. 2011;**1808**(8):1975-1984. DOI: 10.1016 /j.bbamem.2011. 04.012

[182] Conlon JM, Prajeep M, Mechkarska M, Coquet L, Leprince J, Jouenne T, et al. Characterization of the host-defense peptides from skin secretions of Merlin's clawed frog *Pseudhymenochirus Merlini*: Insights into phylogenetic relationships among the Pipidae. Comp. Biochem. Physiol. Part D Genom. Proteonomics. 2013;**8**(4):352-357. DOI: 10.1016/j.cbd.2013.10.002

[183] Ali MF, Soto A, Knoop FC, Conlon JM. Antimicrobial peptides isolated from skin secretions of the diploid frog *Xenopus tropicalis* (Pipidae). Biochimica et Biophysica Acta. 2001;**1550**(1):81-89. DOI: 10.1016/s0167-4838 (01)00272-2

[184] Park CB, Kim MS, Kim SC. A novel antimicrobial peptide from *Bufo bufo*

gargarizans. Biochemical and Biophysical Research Communications. 1996;**218**(1):408-413. DOI: 10. 1006/ bbrc.1996.0071

[185] Fennell JF, Shipman WH, Cole LJ. Antibacterial action of melittin, a polypeptide from bee venom. Proceedings of the Society for Experimental Biology and Medicine. 1968;**127**(3):707-710. DOI: 10.3181/ 00379727-127-32779

[186] Park J, Kwon O, An HJ, Park KK. Antifungal effects of bee venom components on *Trichophyton rubrum*: A novel approach of bee venom study for possible emerging antifungal agent. Annals of Dermatology. 2018;**30**(2):202-210. DOI: 10.5021/ ad.2018.30.2. 202

[187] Pereira AV, de Barros G, Pinto EG, Tempone AG, Orsi RO, Dos Santos LD, et al. Melittin induces *in vitro* death of Leishmania (Leishmania) infantum by triggering the cellular innate immune response. Journal of Venomous Animals and Toxins including Tropical Diseases. 2016;**22**:1. DOI: 10.1186/s40409-016-0055-x

[188] Kim YW, Chaturvedi PK, Chun SN, Lee YG, Ahn WS. Honeybee venom possesses anticancer and antiviral effects by differential inhibition of HPV E6 and E7 expression on cervical cancer cell line. Oncology Reports. 2015;**33**(4): 1675-1682. DOI: 10.3892/or. 2015.3760

[189] Van den Bogaart G, Guzman JV, Mika JT, Poolman B. On the mechanism of pore formation by melittin. The Journal of Biological Chemistry. 2008; **283**(49):33854-33857. DOI: 10.1074/jbc. M805171200

[190] Rangel K, Lechuga GC, Almeida Souza AL, Carvalho JPRS, Villas-Bôas MHS, De Simone SG. Pan-drug resistant Acinetobacter baumannii but not other strains are resistant to the bee venom peptide melittin. Antibiotics (Basel). 2020;**149**(4):178. DOI: 10.3390/ antibiotics9040178

[191] Steiner H, Hultmark D, Engström Å, Bennich H, Boman HG. Sequence and specificity of two antibacterial proteins involved in insect immunity. Nature. 1981;**292**(5820):246. DOI: 10.1038/ 292246a0

[192] Hui L, Leung K, Chen HM. The combined effects of antibacterial peptide cecropin a and anticancer agents on leukemia cells. Anticancer Research. 2002;**22**(5):2811-2816

[193] Wu Q, Patočka J, Kuča K. Insect Antimicrobial Peptides, a Mini Review. Toxins (Basel). 2018;**10**(11):461. DOI: 10.3390/toxins10110461

[194] Yun J, Lee DG. Cecropin A-induced apoptosis is regulated by ion balance and glutathione antioxidant system in *Candida albicans*. IUBMB Life. 2016;**68**(8):652-662. DOI: 10.1002/ iub.1527

[195] Hirai Y, Yasuhara T, Yoshida H, Nakajima T, Fujino M, Kitada C. A new mast cell degranulating peptide "mastoparan" in the venom of *Vespula lewisii*. Chem Pharm Bull (Tokyo). 1979; **27**(8):1942-1944. DOI: 10.1248/ cpb.27.1942

[196] Moreno M, Giralt E. Three valuable peptides from bee and wasp venoms for therapeutic and biotechnological use: Melittin apamin and mastoparan. Toxins. 2015;**7**(4):1126-1150. DOI: 10.3390/toxins7041126

[197] Chen X, Zhang L, Wu Y, Wang L, Ma C, Xi X, et al. Evaluation of the bioactivity of a mastoparan peptide from wasp venom and of its analogues designed through targeted engineering. International Journal of Biological Sciences. 2018;**14**(6):599-607. DOI: 10.7150/ijbs.234 19

[198] Sun H, Hong Y, Xi Y, Zou Y, Gao J, Du J. Synthesis self-assembly and biomedical applications of antimicrobial peptide-polymer conjugates.

Biomacromolecules. 2018;**19**(6):1701-1720. DOI: 10.1021/acs.biomac.8b00 208

[199] Oppenheim FG, Xu T, McMillian FM, Levitz SM, Diamond RD, Offner GD, et al. Histatins a novel family of histidine-rich proteins in human parotid secretion isolation characterization primary structure and fungistatic effects on *Candida albicans*. The Journal of Biological Chemistry. 1988;**263**(16): 7472-7477

[200] Murakami Y, Tamagawa H, Shizukuishi S, Tsunemitsu A, Aimoto S. Biological role of an arginine residue present in a histidine-rich peptide which inhibits hemagglutination of *Porphyromonas gingivalis*. FEMS Microbiology Letters. 1992;**77**(1–3):201-204. DOI: 10.1016/0378-1097(92)90156-i

[201] Burian M, Schittek B. The secrets of dermcidin action. International Journal of Medical Microbiology. 2015; **305**(2):283-286. DOI: 10.1016/j.ijmm.2014.12.012

[202] Muta T, Fujimoto T, Nakajima H, Iwanaga S. Tachyplesins isolated from hemocyte of southeast Asian horseshoe crabs (*Carcinoscorpius rotundicauda* and *Tachypleus gigas*): Identification of a new tachyplesin tachyplesin III and a processing intermediate of its precursor. Journal of Biochemistry. 1990;**108**(9): 261-266. DOI: 10.1093/oxfordjournals.jbchem.a123191

[203] Liu C, Qi J, Shan B, Ma Y. Tachyplesin causes membrane instability that kills multidrug-resistant bacteria by inhibiting the 3-ketoacyl carrier protein reductase FabG. Frontiers in Microbiology. 2018;**9**:825. DOI: 10.3389/fmicb.2018.00825

[204] Rahbar MR, Zarei M, Jahangiri A, Khalili S, Nezafat N, Negahdaripour M, et al. Pierce into the native structure of Ata, a trimeric autotransporter of *Acinetobacter baumannii* ATCC 17978. Int. J. Pept. Res. Therapeut. 2020;**26**: 1269-1282

[205] Jahangiri A, Rasooli I, Owlia P, Fooladi AAI, Salimian J. An integrative in silico approach to the structure of Omp33-36 in *Acinetobacter baumannii*. Computational Biology and Chemistry. 2018;**72**:77-86. DOI: 10.1016/j.compbiolchem.2018.01.003

[206] Rasooli I, Abdolhamidi R, Jahangiri A, Astaneh DAS. Outer membrane protein Oma87 prevents *Acinetobacter baumannii* infection. International Journal of Peptide Research and Therapeutics. 2020;**9**:1-8. DOI: 10.1007/s10989-020-10056-0

[207] Rahbar MR, Zarei M, Jahangiri A, Khalili S, Nezafat N, Negahdaripour M, et al. Trimeric autotransporter adhesins in *Acinetobacter baumannii* coincidental evolution at work. Infection, Genetics and Evolution. 2019;**71**:116-127. DOI: 10.1016/j. meegid.2019.03.023

[208] Nagarajan D, Nagarajan T, Roy N, Kulkarni O, Ravichandran S, Mishra M, et al. The Journal of Biological Chemistry. 2018;**293**(10):3492-3509. DOI: 10.1074/jbc.M117.805499

[209] Misawa T, Goto C, Shibata N, Hirano M, Kikuchi Y, Naito M, et al. Rational design of novel amphipathic antimicrobial peptides focused on the distribution of cationic amino acid residues. Med. Chem. Comm. 2019;**10**(6): 896-900. DOI: 10.1039/c9md0 0166b

[210] Khan MTH. Recent Trends on QSAR in the Pharmaceutical Perceptions. Sharjah, United Arab Emirates: Bentham Science Publishers; 2012. ISBN: 978-1-60805-433-6

[211] Wu X, Wang Z, Li X, Fan Y, He G, Wan Y, et al. In vitro and in vivo activities of antimicrobial peptides developed using an amino acid-based activity prediction method. Antimicrobial Agents and

Chemotherapy. 2014;**58**(9): 5342-5349

[212] Ageitos JM, Sánchez-Pérez A, Calo-Mata P, Villa TG. Antimicrobial peptides (AMPs): Ancient compounds that represent novel weapons in the fight against bacteria. Biochemical Pharmacology. 2017;**133**:117. DOI: 10.1016/j.bcp.2016.09.018

[213] Andersson DI, Hughes D, Kubicek-Sutherland JZ. Mechanisms and consequences of bacterial resistance to antimicrobial peptides. Drug Resistance Updates. 2016;**26**:43-57. DOI: 10.1016/j.drup. 2016.04.002

[214] Moravej H, Moravej Z, Yazdanparast M, Heiat M, Mirhosseini A, Moghaddam MM, et al. Antimicrobial peptides: Features action and their resistance mechanisms in bacteria. Microbial Drug Resistance. 2018;**24**(6):747. DOI: 10.1089/mdr.2017.0392

[215] Joo HS, Fu CI, Otto M. Bacterial strategies of resistance to antimicrobial peptides. Phil. Trans. R. Soc. Lond. B. Biol. Sci. 2016;**371**(1695):20150292. DOI: 10.1098/rstb. 2015.0292

[216] Omardien S, Brul S, Zaat SAJ. Antimicrobial activity of cationic antimicrobial peptides against gram-positive: Current progress made in understanding the mode of action and the response of bacteria. Front. Cell. Develop. Biol. 2016;**4**:111. DOI: 10.3389/fcell.2016.00111

[217] Jeannot K, Bolard A, Plésiat P. Resistance to polymyxins in gram-negative organisms. Int. J. Antimicr Ag. 2017;**49**(5):526-535. DOI: 10.1016/j.ijantimicag.2016. 11.029

[218] Liu YY, Wang Y, Walsh TR, Yi LX, Zhang R, Spencer J, et al. Emergence of plasmid-mediated colistin resistance mechanism MCR-1 in animals and human beings in China: A microbiological and molecular biological study. The Lancet Infectious Diseases. 2016;**16**(2):161-168. DOI: 10.1016/S1473-3099(15)00424-7

[219] Paterson DL, Harris PNA. Colistin resistance: A major breach in our last line of defense. The Lancet Infectious Diseases. 2016;**16**(2):132-133. DOI: 10.1016/S1473-3099(15)00463-6

[220] Macnair CR, Stokes JM, Carfrae LA, Fiebig-Comyn AA, Coombes BK, Mulvey MR, et al. Overcoming mcr-1 mediated colistin resistance with colistin in combination with other antibiotics. Nature Communications. 2018;**9**(1):458. DOI: 10.1038/s41467-018-02875-z

[221] Morita Y, Tomida J, Kawamura Y. MexXY multidrug efflux system of *Pseudomonas aeruginosa*. Frontiers in Microbiology. 2012;**3**:408. DOI: 10.3389/fmicb.2012.00408

[222] Bechinger B, Gorr SU. Antimicrobial peptides: Mechanisms of action and resistance. Journal of Dental Research. 2017;**96**(3):254-260. DOI: 10.1177/0022034516679973

[223] Gheorghe I, Saviuc C, Ciubuca B, Lazar V, Chifiriuc MC. Chapter 8—Nano drug delivery. In: Grumezescu AM, editor. Nanomaterials for Drug Delivery and Therapy. Norwich NY USA: William Andrew Publishing; 2019. pp. 225-244. ISBN: 978-0-12-816505-8

[224] Sun B, Wibowo D, Middelberg APJ, Zhao CX. Cost-effective downstream processing of recombinantly produced pexiganan peptide and its antimicrobial activity. AMB Express. 2018;**8**(1):1-14. DOI: 10.1186/s13568-018-0541-3

[225] Brannon JR, Burk DL, Leclerc JM, Thomassin JL, Portt A, Berghuis AM, et al. Inhibition of outer membrane proteases of the omptin family by aprotinin. Infection and Immunity. 2015;**83**(6):2300-2311. DOI: 10.1128/IAI.00136-15